OLD Is the
NEW
YOUNG

OLD Is the NEW YOUNG

Erickson's® Secrets to Healthy Living

Mark R. Erickson, Matthew J. Narrett, M.D.,
Jacquelyn Kung, D.P.H., and Lisa Davila

life

Guilford, Connecticut
An imprint of The Globe Pequot Press

To buy books in quantity for corporate use
or incentives, call **(800) 962–0973**
or e-mail **premiums@GlobePequot.com**.

gpp®
life

GPP Life is an imprint of The Globe Pequot Press.

Text designer: Sheryl P. Kober
Layout artist: Kim Burdick
Cover designer: Diana Nuhn
Cover photo by Shutterstock

Library of Congress Cataloging-in-Publication Data

Old is the new young : Erickson's secrets to healthy living / Mark R. Erickson . . . [et al.].
    p. cm.
 Includes bibliographical references.
 ISBN 978-0-7627-5011-5
 1. Aging—Prevention. 2. Self-care, Health. I. Erickson, Mark R. II. Erickson Retirement Communities, LLC.
 RA776.75.053 2009
 612.6'7—dc22

                          2009010717

Printed in the United States of America

10 9 8 7 6 5 4 3 2 1

We dedicate this book to our wonderful families,
as well as the greater Erickson family.

Contents

FOREWORD

E. M. Forster described aging as one of life's great paradoxes, calling it a "seductive combination of increased wisdom and decaying powers to which too little intelligence is devoted." People enjoy living but dislike aging, even though they cannot live without aging. Among the great achievements of the past century has been a dramatic increase—thirty years—in life expectancy at birth. Yet rather than celebrations, we hear lamentations about the aging of the population. This thirty-year longevity bonus has not been fully grasped by individuals or society. I have been working in the field of aging for thirty-five years and have been aging for seventy-one years, so let me explain what I mean.

We see a lot of denial about aging. Have you ever noticed how many people say, "I am twenty-nine and holding" or "I may be getting older, but I'll never get old"? Have you looked through the selection of birthday cards for people fifty and older? They do not paint a very positive picture: "You're over the Hill," "Out to Lunch," "Take your birthday suit to the cleaners, it's wrinkled," and so on. I am not against humor, but I do find "old-age jokes" indicative of a mindset that does not understand the many advances we have made in understanding the aging process and its implications for us throughout our increasingly longer lives. Advances in health and other fields have produced an increase in life expectancy and a reduction in the rate of disability among people at all ages. There is still a lot of life to be lived after the traditional "age of retirement." The average life expectancy for people at age sixty-five is twenty years. Many will live into their nineties, and the capabilities of most of these people are impressive.

I have had the opportunity to work with and know people in their sixties, seventies, eighties, and nineties who are still active, knowledgeable, and contributing to society in many ways. Unfortunately, there are many more who could do so but are prevented by policies, practices, and perceptions. The policies and practices can include mandatory retirement and various forms of age discrimination. By perceptions I mean buying into the negative myths and stereotypes of aging. These perceptions are most harmful when people accept them as they get older, who feel they can't try or learn new things because they are too old. How many of you, when you were children, were told to "act your age"? How many of you have been told by your children to "act your age"? Where is the rulebook? There are books on what to expect of your newborn, your toddler, your preadolescent, and your teen. No one has written a book on what to expect as a middle–age or older adult. How exactly should we act at fifty, sixty, seventy, or any age? There really are no limits as long as you want to do it and your health does not prevent it.

It was something of a surprise some years ago when we learned that exercise was so beneficial to health at all ages. For so long it had been assumed that after a certain age, we should "take it easy." It was even more surprising when studies revealed that lifting weights would increase bone density and muscle mass in people regardless of their age—this is very important in preventing osteoporosis and falls. Like everyone else, I had thought for years that our brains were hard-wired at an early age and then could not change. The discoveries in the past twenty years about brain "plasticity" have shown that with proper stimulation, our brains can rewire themselves at any age. So much for the ridiculous saying, "You can't teach an old dog new tricks." (Actually, it is not even true about dogs.)

We thought for years that genetic makeup totally determined how we age. This explains why people were told that to have an active and vital old age, they should choose their parents carefully. This is not particularly helpful, and, in fact, is not accurate. We now know that our own behavior is responsible for most of how we age. According to a ten-year multidisciplinary study funded by the MacArthur Foundation, the real formula for successful aging consists of disease avoidance, exercise of mind and body, and staying involved in life. Since these points are discussed later in this book, I won't elaborate on them here except to say that some medical experts claim that two-thirds of our health problems are caused by our own behavior.

While the increase in life expectancy and vitality is welcome news, it does present a bigger challenge for people planning for and living in retirement. That challenge is how to make sure you do not outlive your financial assets. Using the age of sixty-five for normal retirement may have been fine when average life expectancy was less than fifty. In such a setting, few retirees lived for many years beyond sixty-five. Now, life expectancy is twenty years on average for people age sixty-five. It takes a lot more planning to arrange for sufficient funds to live that long, and that challenge has become even more complex in recent years.

The traditional formula for providing retirement income was compared to a three-legged stool: Social Security, private pensions, and personal savings. With changes from defined benefit plans to defined contribution plans, savings and private pensions have really become pretty much the same. The new approach for retirement planning consists of four pillars: Social Security, personal savings (including IRAs and 401Ks), health insurance, and earned income. This shift can be especially hard for people in or near retirement, and the state of the economy today has only made it worse.

The bottom line is that the responsibility for our financial security and health insurance is more than ever falling on us—defined benefit pensions are rapidly disappearing, and more of the decisions and costs of our health care are ours as well. Unfortunately, many middle–aged and older people are not well prepared for this and are confused by the choices and decisions before them. Books such as this one and the resources listed in the appendix are very important tools to help us meet the challenge.

I recommend that you read this book and get familiar with its contents. Then, use it as a handy reference tool when needs or questions arise. There are many valuable suggestions contained throughout. Finally, I want to commend Erickson for producing and making this book available and to acknowledge its leadership in promoting healthy aging for its residents, and with this book, the wider population. In doing so, Erickson continues to show the way.

—Horace B. Deets
Board Chair, Longevity Alliance
Board Member, PositScience
Former Executive Director, AARP

Starting a New Chapter in Your Life

Jack[1] is a seventy-five-year-old who retired in his early sixties after a long and lucrative career as a lawyer. He had always enjoyed good health and stayed quite active the first few years, indulging his love of cooking by working part-time for a gourmet caterer and whipping up tasty delicacies for his friends and family at home. In addition, Jack spent a lot of time getting back to his artistic roots—nature photography and playing classical guitar.

After Jack turned seventy, however, he began to change. He lost several close friends and went out less. He gradually stopped working and stopped taking pictures and playing the guitar because of arthritis. Jack's normally adventurous spirit and sense of humor also declined as he became more dependent on his daily routines and resisted trying new activities. To make matters worse, he had always mistrusted doctors and didn't consistently follow prescribed medical advice. To his family, Jack now seemed like the stereotypical old man—isolated, with increasingly failing memory and health and high resistance to change or improvement.

---

[1] *Throughout this book, names and personal details have been changed to protect privacy.*

Helen is also seventy-five. After a lifelong career as a high school teacher, she retired at the age of sixty. The first years of her retirement were spent caring for her ailing mother, who endured a series of debilitating strokes before finally succumbing to a major stroke five years later. After her mother died, Helen decided that she didn't want to suffer the same fate.

Helen had enjoyed good health throughout her life but as she got older developed high cholesterol and became somewhat overweight. She consulted with her doctor and began exercising regularly and eating a healthy diet. Helen's cholesterol profile improved greatly, and her weight came down. She felt better physically, had more energy, and had a sense of pride in her accomplishments.

Along with a healthy body, Helen also wanted to keep her mind sharp—something she valued greatly as a former teacher. She noticed gradual, minor memory lapses and realized that her daily crossword puzzles were probably not enough to stimulate her brain. She decided to get more involved in her church by trying some new things—singing in the choir and organizing outings for various church groups. Now Helen feels mentally sharper and her family has noticed that she's happy, relaxed, and looks better than ever.

When you think about retirement, would you rather be like Jack or Helen? Do you feel a foreboding sense of dread or do you envision this period of your life as an exciting opportunity for new adventures? You may have preconceived fears that your retirement years mean inevitable decline and boredom. You may think you have to endure activities like bridge and bingo, wheelchairs for transportation, or the eventual loss of your individuality in an institutional setting if your health worsens.

Good news! This clichéd description of retirement no longer applies. Today's active seniors play pickle ball and

Nintendo Wii instead of bingo. They start walking groups instead of using wheelchairs. They sing popular and rock music in choral groups. Today's seniors are able to do so much because major treatment advancements for conditions like heart disease, diabetes, and cancer mean that older Americans can expect to live longer and enjoy more active lifestyles than previous generations.

You can remain informed, inspired, and involved in life with just a few small investments in your health. Investing in your health means engaging in preventive health care practices like exercising and eating the right foods. These investments can be especially beneficial as you get older because, although you may seem to age at a faster rate each passing year, your body is very forgiving. You have the power to slow down some aging processes and change some negatives to positives.

How do we know this is possible? Because we are Erickson, and our twenty-five years of experience in the retirement industry has given us unique knowledge and perspectives about aging successfully.

The Erickson Mission—One Man's Vision

John Erickson, founder and CEO of Erickson, has a deep passion for challenging the old concepts of retirement. In the early years of his career, he managed mobile-home communities in Florida. He witnessed firsthand the inactive, stilted existence of many seniors and set out to create a different type of retirement—one that embodied a vibrant and active lifestyle.

It seemed like a simple idea: Create an environment where people not only have fun, but also where the emphasis is on maintaining one's best health. John Erickson put his plan into motion in the early 1980s with the purchase of a hundred-acre abandoned theological college campus in Baltimore. The first Erickson continuing care retirement community opened, and its pioneering residents got to experience a more active lifestyle than they ever dreamed possible—an even more stimulating environment for some residents than their college days.

Traditional continuing care retirement communities offer various levels of living assistance and services for seniors. Erickson communities, however, are dynamic social environments that give their members unlimited opportunities to remain actively involved yet are also designed to respect and protect each individual's privacy. Erickson residents live comfortably in spacious apartments, dine in on-campus restaurants with a variety of menus, learn new skills in creative arts studios and computer labs, and involve themselves in interesting activities and lectures—all while maintaining their best health possible with on-campus physicians and close ties to family and the surrounding community.

Now with twenty communities nationwide and growing, John Erickson continues to change society's pervasive but archaic views about aging and retirement. Profiled in the *Wall Street Journal* as an innovator and leader for aging in America, John Erickson leads with a simple message to all Erickson employees and residents: Share your gifts to create communities that celebrate life.

Why Erickson Living?

Erickson Living is our philosophy at Erickson Retirement Communities. Why? Because although the word "retirement" is often viewed positively—evoking thoughts of freedom and leisure, and the word "community" connotes a place where people connect, care about each other, interact, and engage. But put these two positive words together, and it triggers the negative image of a nursing home. "Living," on the other hand, is much more descriptive of the choices and attitudes of Erickson residents.

Residents who choose the Erickson lifestyle spend between one-fourth to one-half less time in hospitals compared to their peers. Why? Because of their engagement with life and our outstanding health care system. Erickson Living creates an engaging lifestyle—a place where people can add more life to their years.

The Erickson Corporation —a Leading Authority on Aging

Erickson is recognized as a leader in senior living, research, education, health care, media, philanthropy, and addressing issues important to seniors and society. Erickson is a major resource for the government, leading research institutions, and worldwide experts on aging. We answer questions about public policy, partner with researchers on cutting-edge health and wellness interventions, and host experts from around the world who want to learn about the best practices in healthy aging.

The Erickson Foundation

The Foundation invests millions of dollars in cutting-edge aging research that has resulted in exciting findings about memory fitness and physical health. Collaborating with the Center on Aging at University of California, Los Angeles, Erickson Foundation researchers found that older adults' memories were enhanced following a six-week program focusing on memory training, physical activity, stress reduction, and dietary teaching. Several additional ongoing studies with regard to memory enhancement show promising preliminary results.

The Foundation's Research and Development program focuses primarily on projects designed to enhance practical knowledge relevant to advancing current best practices in support of the health care, educational, social, residential, emotional, and spiritual needs of mature adults. For example, the Erickson Life Study evaluates residents over the long term with regard to changes in health status and which community amenities and services they use. The Community Mobility and Safe Driving Program conducted studies focused on tools to evaluate older drivers' safe driving capacity. The program is now piloting a driver safety education program for seniors. The Foundation's research priorities are understanding older adults' strengths, needs, and preferences; enabling healthy choices and pursuits; preserving and enhancing wellness; preventing disease and disability; and building partnership opportunities.

The Erickson School of Aging, Management and Policy
Located at the University of Maryland's Baltimore County campus, the Erickson School provides undergraduate and graduate degrees and executive education—all with an explicit focus on educating a community of leaders who will improve society by enhancing the lives of older adults. The Erickson School's mission is to inspire change and help reinvent the way society views and responds to aging.

Housed within the Erickson School is the Center for Aging Studies, which is the hub for Erickson's faculty and student research. A multidisciplinary team of researchers representing anthropology, sociology, health services and aging services research, and gerontology are at the Center's core. Striving to enhance the well-being of elderly people, the Center works collaboratively with professionals, policy makers, researchers, and service practitioners in the field of aging by sharing research findings and developing new research and demonstration projects that deal with real issues, like seniors' health care and housing.

Led by Erickson School faculty member Dr. Bill Thomas, researchers developed the Green House Model, a radically new approach to long-term care in which traditional nursing homes are replaced with small, home-like environments where people can live a full and interactive life. Partially funded by the Robert Wood Johnson Foundation, Green House projects are being launched in all fifty states.

Erickson Health

As the nation's largest integrated health and wellness system for older adults, this unique network of health care professionals includes physicians, nurses, therapists, social workers, and other staff who make use of a highly coordinated network of health care services, information, research, and electronic medical records to provide top-notch care to Erickson residents. What started as a one-man physician practice has grown into Erickson Health Medical Group, the nation's largest physician practice whose sole focus is older adults' health and wellness.

Older adults' health needs are different from their younger counterparts—often becoming progressively complicated by mounting health conditions, multiple medications, and functional limitations related to aging. Erickson Health doctors address not only medical aspects of their patients' care, but also psychological, social, and functional aspects. Because an interdisciplinary approach is essential to providing coordinated and seamless services, Erickson Health doctors work closely with nurse practitioners, psychiatrists, surgical specialists, podiatrists, pharmacists, social workers, and physical and occupational therapists to ensure the best care for their patients. Erickson Health is now also being offered to older adults living outside of Erickson communities.

Retirement Living TV

The country's first television network for older Americans was launched by John Erickson to change society's commonly held, often erroneous views about older adults. Retirement Living TV is the new voice of a generation underserved by the media industry and features a variety of shows addressing important senior social and health issues. *The Daily Café* has the latest news and trends affecting viewers age fifty-five and older, tackling subjects ranging from caregiving to managing your nest egg. *Healthline* offers up-to-the-minute health information and personal stories. *Retired and Wired* is a guide to the latest high-tech tips and tools that teaches viewers how to make technology work for them. By combining original programming with public affairs campaigns, partnerships, and resources, Retirement Living TV raises awareness and encourages discourse on these important issues for seniors, caregivers, and families alike. Check your local listings to tune in.

For more information about The Erickson Foundation's research, The Erickson School of Aging's programs, Erickson Health's services, or Retirement Living TV, see Appendix B.

Your Secrets for Healthy Living

What does "aging successfully" mean to you? Our research shows that successful aging means maintaining your health, activity level, and independence. It also means staying happy, mentally alert, and socially active. Getting started means taking control of your health—doing this now will improve your chances of remaining independent.

We at Erickson have been studying the aging process and serving the needs of seniors across the nation for twenty-five years. We will share with you the ten secrets we have discovered during this journey. We will highlight these secrets by talking about our experiences over the years and sharing examples from our residents. We will review research and dispel myths along the way. We will offer assessments so you can test yourself in some areas. And we will offer recommendations and tips—things that you can start doing today to improve your aging process.

There are really two parts to successful aging: The first is having the right information; the second is making the right choices. This book will give you all the information you need to age successfully. But ultimately, it's up to you to act on the right choices.

CHAPTER ONE

Take Control of Your Health Now for More Independence Later

"Every man desires to live long, but no man would be old."

—Jonathan Swift, *Thoughts on Various Subjects* (1711)

As former baseball great Satchel Paige once asked, "How old would you be if you didn't know your age?" Today, most people over age fifty would probably say that they feel ten to twenty years younger. If fifty is the new forty, then seventy is the new sixty, right? Your older years are the perfect time to become informed, inspired, and involved in life—in other words, to be young again. Better health care has given you extended longevity, and you have both the opportunity and the freedom to have a different and better second half of life. The kids have grown and you've worked hard all of your life. Your retirement years can now mark a time when you get to try new things—perhaps even some activities you have longed to do for much of your life but never felt you had the time.

Realizing an opportunity for a new youth is not easy for everyone, as aging often comes with some physical and cognitive limitations. We at Erickson know about these limitations, but we can still help you age successfully. Through our experiences, we have discovered the secrets behind healthy aging, which we share throughout this book. If you want to live a better, longer life, then you want your later years to be healthy and fulfilling. You need to know what to do now to ensure a better future. In this book, we focus on four key areas of life fitness: physical, mental, social, and financial. In each of these areas, we'll show you how to keep what you have, get back what you've lost, and tap into your natural resiliency by compensating when necessary.

Your body and mind have tremendous reserve and potential even well into advancing age. You can make the upcoming years the best they can be. Old is the new young. Start your new life now.

You're Living Longer in Good Company

Of all retirement-age adults who have ever lived, half are alive today. That means you have plenty of company as you enter your retirement years. So think of these years as your second half of life, a new beginning and a great time to make changes for the better—because you and your peers are living longer than ever.

In the early 1900s, the average life expectancy was about fifty years. By 1950, it had increased to seventy years, and today, most adults can expect to live about eighty years. There has never been a better time to be alive because of modern medicine and new technologies. A hundred years ago, for example, it wasn't possible to implant a pacemaker in someone whose heart rhythm needed regulating. Today it is possible, and many heart patients are healthier and live longer.

Longer life expectancies mean an ever-growing older population. The U.S. Census reports that Clearwater, Florida, has the highest percentage of adults over age sixty-five—a full 22 percent of its 110,000 population. Cape Coral, Florida, comes in second with about 20 percent of its 100,000 population in their retirement years. Overall, about 17 percent of Florida's entire population is age sixty-five and over (West Virginia is second with 15.5 percent, and Pennsylvania is third with 15.2 percent). By 2030, the entire country will be like Clearwater, with about one out of every five people qualifying for Medicare.

Because more of your life will be lived during your retirement years, you need to have a plan to make those years healthier and happier. We'll help you develop that plan. In addition to covering the four most important areas in your life—physical, mental, social, and financial—throughout the book we'll also share with you our "secrets" for successful aging. And while separately each of these life lessons may seem obvious at first, when you pull them all together and truly follow each one, you'll have a real road map for keeping the *freedom* in your freedom years.

Secret #1: It *Can* Be Done

As George Burns once said, "You can't help getting older, but you can help getting old." That's right—getting older doesn't mean getting *old*. Our societal values have trained us to believe that aging is associated with unavoidable decline and disability. This is simply not the case. Because you have the power to make changes that will keep you informed, involved, and inspired by life, you have the power to feel younger.

Helping yourself to avoid "getting old" can be done. It involves some common sense and a few small investments in your body, mind, social network, and finances. But first, you need to identify your strengths and weaknesses. Enlist the aid of your doctor, your family and friends, people from your community groups and place of worship, and your financial advisor. Once you've done your self-assessment, you can formulate a plan for improvement. And despite commonly held misconceptions, the rewards can come quickly. You'll see in some of the following examples how simple, manageable changes can make a tremendous difference.

Small Changes Can Lead to Big Improvements

Lorraine is a sixty-three-year-old who didn't walk a lot and primarily used a scooter to get around. She felt somewhat depressed about the aging process because she had problems performing her daily activities. She opted to participate in the Erickson Foundation's Viva! program, which is a comprehensive health and wellness screening that evaluates physical, psychological, and social factors. After her assessment, Lorraine was disgusted with her low scores in several areas and was determined to change them.

She began by walking a little more each day, measuring her steps with a pedometer to keep track of her progress. She started taking tai chi classes to improve her balance and strength. She also became more involved in her community so that she wouldn't feel so isolated.

Lorraine returned one year later for a follow-up assessment. She had tripled her step count, her body fat composition dropped by 5 percent, she reported few functional difficulties, and she had little need for her scooter. In addition, Lorraine's depression scores improved and she reported a renewed sense of satisfaction with life.

Simple Steps to a Healthy Lifestyle

Throughout her life, seventy-year-old Laura had been outgoing and enjoyed socializing. After retiring from her job at an international bank, she knew keeping active would be important for her continued good health. When she and her husband moved into an Erickson community, she started going to the fitness center. But after a while, Laura found herself involved in so many activities that she didn't have as much time for the fitness center. To compensate, she began walking to all of her activities, and then walking some more.

Laura believes that being involved in the Asian club, yoga, and the weekly "treasure sale" (in which Erickson residents sell their extra furniture, clothing, and so on, to benefit other residents who need financial support) helps her stay both physically healthy and mentally sharp.

Regarding her diet, Laura keeps it simple: She avoids fatty foods except for the occasional splurge. Laura says that keeping healthy is easy—do what's good for you and makes you happy. For her that means a lot of walking, socializing, and eating a low-fat diet.

Starting from Scratch Financially—One Dollar at a Time
Diane was in her mid-fifties when she went through a difficult divorce—leaving her with no house and little money. Initially, she felt hopeless because her only income came from teaching organ lessons and playing at her local church.

Instead of becoming depressed, Diane decided to view her situation as an opportunity to try something new. She applied for a job at a temp agency and eventually got placed in over a dozen jobs. Several employers even offered her full-time positions. After accepting one of the full-time offers, Diane looked into buying a house. She asked her boss's advice and found a mortgage agent she trusted.

Diane learned what she could afford and purchased a home. But she didn't have enough money to furnish it—all she owned was a bed and a small table. Rather than borrowing money, Diane gradually put aside whatever she could from her earnings and bought one piece of furniture at a time. Eventually she completely furnished her home, and she didn't go into debt to do it.

Now over twenty years later, Diane has remarried and has sold her house for twice its original value. Diane says the secret to rebuilding her life was to keep moving forward and not to let anything overwhelm her.

Secret #2: Think Positively

You may have noticed that our residents' stories share a common theme: Each individual had the motivation to make life changes in large part because they were thinking positively. You might think as you go through your retirement years that you will develop a pessimistic, "crotchety" attitude. You are basing this thinking, no doubt, on society's pervasive stereotype of the lonely and crusty older adult. And it's true that a recent Tufts University study found that older people were often dubbed "grouchy," "lonely," and "weak."

But one of the longest-running studies about aging has found that these stereotypes are simply *not* true. A group of over one hundred scientists involved in the Baltimore Longitudinal Study have found that personalities remain essentially unchanged as we age.

This personality theory is not new. Carl Jung, the great psychiatrist and founder of analytical psychology, believed that we are born with certain personality traits and temperaments that don't change. These are the *predispositions* to our personalities. He also believed, however, that as we mature we acquire character—a set of habits that becomes our actual *disposition*. So just because you're born with a certain personality doesn't mean that you can't change some aspects of it.

A recent groundbreaking thirty-year study published by sociologists at the University of Chicago showed that among adults ages eighteen to eighty-eight, older adults were happier than their younger counterparts. In fact, the odds of being happy increased by 5 percent every ten years. This study affirms Jung's theories that with maturity comes the development of positive changes—like increased self-esteem—that lead to an overall feeling of happiness and contentment. And, as we age, we tend to lower our expectations of ourselves, which generally leads to a higher level of satisfaction and overall happiness.

You now have a good reason to think positively: The societal myth about age equating to unhappiness has been dispelled through extensive research.

Thinking Positively: Expectations versus Satisfaction

Professor Tom DeLong of Harvard Business School teaches that satisfaction equals what you achieve divided by what you expect. In other words, if you have low expectations but have the exact same results as if you had high expectations, your satisfaction level will be higher. For example, think about the last time you went to a movie that you didn't expect to like, but after seeing it you really enjoyed it and felt very satisfied that you went. If you had high expectations for that movie, you would have walked out of the theater thinking it simply met your expectations and would not have felt nearly as satisfied.

Lowering your expectations does not necessarily mean that you have to do less. In fact, when it comes to social activities, the University of Chicago study showed that people in their eighties tend to participate in twice the social activities as their retiree counterparts in their fifties. Lowering your expectations means that you learn to appreciate yourself and the things you do every day without expecting perfect results.

Learning Optimism

Why should you bother to learn how to be optimistic? Because positive attitudes help you become strong and resilient as you age. Can you learn to think positively if you were born with a predisposition to pessimism? Experts think so.

World-renowned psychologist Martin Seligman noticed a phenomenon called "learned helplessness" while experimenting with animals. He noticed that some dogs became dejected after failing during an experiment. Their performance on subsequent experiments was even worse, and they became more despondent.

Seligman noticed this same behavior in people. After failing an endeavor, some people convince themselves that they can't try again. Seligman noticed that people in this state of mind not only felt like they couldn't perform a failed task again but also thought they wouldn't be able to perform an unrelated task. This state of mind resulted in a downward emotional spiral.

Fortunately, Seligman also noticed a phenomenon called "learned optimism," whereby people can encourage themselves and succeed at a previously failed task. It's not that optimists don't fail; it's just that they're able to brush off failure as a temporary circumstance and focus on their next goal. They're resilient.

Harvard psychotherapist and aging expert Dr. Terry Bard argues that even if you are pessimistic by nature, you can learn the behaviors that will help you have an optimistic outlook. A positive attitude that helps you get through daily life trials is not generic, run-of-the-mill optimism. Rather, it's about adopting a different way of interpreting events: Failures are not linked to character flaws, and successes are not a matter of sheer good luck. In addition, a series of Harvard research studies has indicated that optimists enjoy better health than pessimists, possibly due in part to healthier lifestyle choices and stronger support networks.

Tips for Thinking Positively

Learning to think positively is a valuable skill that can help you adapt to life's daily struggles. We don't pretend that positive thinking will cure everything, but a positive, proactive attitude is critical for successful aging. Even if you think you've had more than your share of hardships, you can still learn to practice the art of thinking positively, as the following tips and examples illustrate.

Tip #1: Compare your situation with someone who has it worse.

In other words, be (or at least act) thankful for what you have. Some of our most optimistic and resilient Erickson customers, despite having several health conditions or having experienced multiple losses in their lives, remain thankful for their current situations because they can always find someone who has it worse.

Eighty-six-year-old Ted, a former military officer, is a tall man with a booming voice. Plagued with a number of serious medical problems, he can only comfortably get around with the help of a motorized scooter and needs some assistance with simple daily tasks. Yet Ted is always laughing and joking with others, and he enjoys the good food and camaraderie at his daily lunches with friends. When asked how he stays so positive and resilient given his limitations, he says, "I have it good. When I look around, I can always find someone who's doing worse than me." From across the table, his friend Frank, age eighty-three, agrees: "So much more could be wrong. We really do have it good."

Ted and Frank are grateful for what they have, and that gives them a positive outlook on life. Instead of focusing on their challenges, they choose to foster a sense of gratitude for the many things they have to be thankful for.

Tip #2: Change your negative thoughts when something bad happens.

In any bad situation, try to find a positive thought or explanation for what happened. Don't allow yourself to get caught up in a negative downward spiral; instead, do your best to accept the situation and focus on what brings you joy—however small it may be.

Karen is a petite, pleasant, seventy-eight-year-old woman who was diagnosed eight years ago with benign vocal cord tumors that required surgery. At about the same time, she began showing signs of macular degeneration, a disease characterized by a gradual loss of central vision.

After her vocal cord operation, Karen needed months of speech therapy to bring her voice up to an audible, yet broken croak. She lost many friends, who told her that they could not tolerate the sound of her voice. At the same time, Karen's vision deteriorated, and she could not clearly see people who were talking to her or items on grocery store shelves. Even watching television became a burden—she had to turn her head and strain to see the screen using her peripheral vision.

Karen became depressed because of all she'd lost—her voice, vision, and many friends. She frequently had negative thoughts. To make herself feel better, Karen started thinking about what she still had—a loving family, a few true friends, good health otherwise, and a wonderful home. She was able to change her thinking about her losses. She realized that friends who disappear because of how your voice sounds are friends not worth having. She could still go out shopping and enjoy other activities because there were people and devices available to help her with her declining vision. Today, Karen is happier and more active than ever because she changed her negative thinking.

Tip #3: Make an effort to smile.

Walk around with a smile or pleasant expression on your face. Watch how others react. Think about how it makes you feel when someone smiles at you. A positive attitude is contagious—the more you walk around with a smile and a sense of optimism, the more likely that feeling will grow and affect others around you.

Rose grew up in the southern United States, where she endured both frank and subtle bigotry for much of her life. As a child, she attended school with other black children and was not allowed to go to certain restaurants or ride freely on buses.

Rose eventually became a nurse and cared for thousands of people in the hospital during her long career. Many people who meet her comment that Rose, who is now ninety-two, has one of the brightest smiles and best attitudes they've ever seen. In fact, one friend describes her smiles as cookies—you get one and feel better right away.

Despite her rough childhood and numerous personal losses over the years—including her sister to cancer and her husband to Alzheimer's disease—Rose is able to maintain a positive attitude. She explains, "I always look forward to tomorrow because it's a brand new day. My mother always told me that I was special and had worth. And she was right. I feel good about myself and want to share my joy with others, so I keep on smiling!"

Secret #3: Care for Yourself

By now you should recognize that you do have the ability to determine the quality of some of your life experiences as you age. While some say that genes are the most important factor for living a long, healthy life, we disagree. In fact, researchers have found that improvements in lifestyles and attitudes pertaining to the four key areas of life—physical, mental, social, and financial—are as important if not more so than your genetic makeup.

A lengthy study looked at approximately six thousand London civil service workers and found that factors such as healthy lifestyles (including good diets, exercise, and no tobacco), along with lower stress levels and an active social network, were more important in determining successful aging than genes. In many U.S. studies, a healthy lifestyle has been shown to decrease the risk of many age-associated diseases like heart disease and diabetes.

A different study, however, found that less than 4 percent of adults consistently follow healthy lifestyle characteristics such as not smoking, eating fruits and vegetables, maintaining a healthy body weight, and engaging in physical activity.

Throughout your life you may have focused on caring for others—your kids, other relatives, and friends. And in your working life you took care of business. But now it's time to take care of yourself. Making small investments in your four crucial life areas can lead to more independence later.

You can find information about healthy aging everywhere—magazines, books, television, the Internet. What can you do when so many experts and scientific findings contradict one another? Should you take a multivitamin? Can daily crossword puzzles keep your brain sharp? Should you buy long-term care insurance?

Our goal is to share our extensive research on physical, mental, social, and financial health with our practical experience keeping Erickson residents healthy. We'll present you with the simplest, most helpful things you and your loved ones can do to stay active and engaged with life.

Your Body

Having a larger population living longer means that people are staying healthier longer than ever. Cancer, heart disease, and strokes used to commonly take their toll on people before they were age 60. If people lived to age seventy, they were likely to be disabled and often in need of a nursing home. But advancements in preventing and treating diseases have allowed us as a population to lead more active lives—right until our time is up.

Since 1900, improvements in public health, vaccinations, and medical care in general have minimized the risk of contracting diseases like tuberculosis or smallpox. But as you age in today's world, you may develop chronic health conditions, which can vary in severity but are persistent and most likely will affect you for the rest of your life. These include arthritis, dementia, diabetes, and heart, lung, or other diseases affecting your major organs. Nearly half of the U.S. population has at least one, and more than 60 percent of those over age sixty-five have more than one of these conditions. Moreover, 25 percent of people with one or more chronic health conditions have limitations in their daily functional activities. The amount of disability increases with the number of chronic health conditions and, not surprisingly, increases your health care utilization, decreases your overall quality of life, and increases your chances of death.

The secrets to living a functional and independent life in your older years are found in lifestyle improvements and reducing your risk of developing a chronic health condition, but also managing it well once you have one. To accomplish these goals you have to make good lifestyle choices, like those pertaining to fitness and diet. We'll tell you how and why in Chapter Two.

Your Brain

When is the last time you forgot where you put your keys? Does it seem to happen more often as you get older? Is declining memory inevitable as you age?

Until the 1980s scientists believed that we lost brain cells (up to a million a day!) as we aged. As technology has improved, however, research shows that there is no relationship between age and total number of brain cells.

What changes as you age are the *connections* between brain cells. These connections help facilitate mental processing but slow down with the aging process. In addition, there are declines in certain brain chemicals that affect these connections. The good news is that long-term knowledge acquired over a lifetime and certain kinds of memory stay largely intact.

Even better news is that you have some power to change this slowing-down process, which often occurs because of a slowed-down lifestyle. We'll tell you how in Chapter Three.

Your Social Life

A popular misconception about older adults is that they are lonely and have lower levels of happiness and satisfaction, or that they have fewer social contacts because careers have slowed down or stopped and children have moved out. Happiness experts disagree. They claim that enduring happiness comes from reaching for specific goals and achievements, and although your goals may change as you age, you can still formulate new ones that fit your lifestyle. And social contacts? The University of Chicago happiness study showed that three out of four adults ages fifty-seven to eighty-five participate in at least one social activity per week, and many have more good friends and better family relationships than younger adults.

Some older adults' social networks decrease, however, when they lose their spouse or close friends. In Chapter Four, we'll show you how to build or maintain your social support network.

Your Financial Picture

A 2006 national survey conducted by Erickson showed that older voters do not want to hear about endless solutions concerning Medicare and Social Security. They want to know how to receive better health care services, better education for children and grandchildren, and lower living costs for themselves and their families. But in spite of these concerns, less than half of Americans admit to having a solid financial plan for their retirement years.

Financial well-being is a topic in this book primarily because money enables you to invest in yourself and live independently. Although the best things in life are free—spending time with family and friends, watching the sunset—you still need money to put healthy food on the table and to help you stay active, both physically and socially.

Staying healthy financially starts with a brief discussion about fixed incomes, Social Security, and Medicare. By some estimates, if our government doesn't make changes, Social Security will be in trouble by 2041 and Medicare by 2019, or even earlier. This means that you have to make smart investments to ensure continued health and well-being. In Chapter Five we'll tell you how.

How All the Pieces Fit: Older Adult Achievers

Bob is eighty-two years old and has completed forty-two marathons. He hasn't been running his whole life, but in fact started at age forty-five when he noticed he was putting on some weight. He started simply, by running up and down the street, keeping track of his mileage. Then he found a group of men to jog with on Saturdays. The group began running in some short races, and eventually they formed a club to run together in longer races.

Bob is not only a marathon runner but a triathlete. His workouts maintain and improve his physical well-being as well as keep him mentally and socially fit. He ran with the club until he moved to another state, where he now enjoys exercising at a gym as well as bicycling with his son once a week. His active lifestyle keeps his medical and prescription bills down. Bob's financial soundness means he can buy new running shoes when necessary and even take his buddies out for a drink once in a while.

Bob may be exceptional, but he's not the only example of an older adult who has remained actively engaged in life well into maturity. At age seventy-two years and 222 days, Japan's Yuichira Miura was the oldest man to scale Mount Everest. In 2008, seventy-two-year-old grandmother Iloo Gruder led a thirteen-person team to a 14,000-foot Himalayan summit in Bhutan to raise money for the treatment of multiple sclerosis and Parkinson's disease. The United States is home to Doug Crary, a tennis champ in his nineties, Charin Yuthasastrkosol, a ballerina in her seventies, Elliot Carter, a one-hundred-year-old composer of classical music, and James Hylton, a race car driver in his seventies aiming to qualify for NASCAR. There's Jack LaLanne, the pioneering fitness, exercise, and nutrition expert, still going strong in his nineties. And many are familiar with the work of Anna Mary Robertson Moses (better known as Grandma Moses), who began painting in her seventies after abandoning a career in embroidery because of arthritis. She lived to be over one hundred.

Right here at Erickson communities we have many seniors who don't fit society's retiree stereotypes. Anne, who is 101 years old, tutors immigrants in English, grows vegetables in her garden, and gives tours to prospective Erickson residents. Jean, who is over ninety, regularly drives to her job at a real estate company across town.

A significant majority of people over fifty, sixty, and even the traditional retirement age of sixty-five, still work. In fact, these statistics led the American Association of Retired Persons to reconsider its name. A full two-thirds of AARP members work, so they now call themselves "the organization formerly known as the American Association of Retired Persons."

Getting Started: Rate Yourself

How do you rate your health compared to other people your age? Is it excellent, good, fair, or poor? This question may seem pointless, but research shows that your honest answers may correlate closely with your actual health status and may even be a predictor of your mortality. You can rate yourself based on your physical condition, daily living activities, mental functioning, emotional status, and social functioning. Your answers can give you clues about where you need improvements.

We've created a simple assessment to help you determine how best to use this book.

RATE YOURSELF
How would you rate your overall health at the present time?

A. excellent
B. good
C. okay
D. fair
E. poor

How is your present health compared to five years ago?
A. much better
B. somewhat better
C. the same
D. somewhat worse
E. much worse

Has your health interfered with things you want to do?
A. no, not at all
B. no, but I can't seem to do as much
C. yes, a small amount
D. yes, a moderate amount
E. yes, a great deal

Give yourself five points for each A, four points for each B, three points for each C, two points for each D, and one point for each E. Add your total points for all three questions.

If you scored 12–15 points, you should aim to maintain your good health and keep what you've got. If you scored 5–11 points, you should look to maintain what you've got and get back some of what you've lost. If you scored 0–4 points, work on building your resiliency and finding ways to make your life easier.

Along with our assessment, there are several longevity and life-expectancy calculators available to help you assess your current lifestyle and its effects on the quality of your retirement years. See Appendix A for examples.

Now that you've rated your health, you can identify what you need to change. Take control of the four areas of your life: physical, mental, social, and financial. Use our tips and experience to map out a road to healthier, happier retirement years, beginning with improving your physical health through diet, exercise, and other preventive measures.

CHAPTER TWO

Keep Your Body Young

"If I'd known I was going to live so long, I'd have taken better care of myself."

—Leon Eldred

Although it may seem that everything in your body is decreasing, drooping, or dropping, your body has more resiliency than you might think. There are many aspects of the physical aging process that are preventable or even reversible. Age may be all in your mind, but only you can keep it from adversely affecting your body.

In this chapter you'll learn how to keep what you have, get back what you can, and how to compensate when necessary when it comes to your physical health.

Facts about Your Aging Body

Not millions or billions, but trillions. That's how many cells you have in your body—more than 4.6 trillion, in fact. That's more than the number of stars in our galaxy. Each cell is a certain type, like skin cells, liver cells, blood cells, and so on. Most of your cells reproduce and replace themselves throughout your lifetime (but only to a certain degree), and then the replication process slows down. And certain types of cells, like your brain and heart cells, are present from birth, grow to maturity, and replicate very slowly if at all.

This replication slowdown means that as early as your late twenties and early thirties, your muscle mass and bone density start decreasing. This decrease in mass is measurable: You actually begin shrinking at a rate of about one-sixteenth of an inch per year starting at age forty. No wonder some people gasp at being two inches shorter when measured at age seventy. Your weight, however, tends to increase until your mid-fifties, when it starts to decline. That's because beginning at about age thirty, your body burns approximately twelve fewer calories per day. What's more, assuming you have similar diet and exercise habits as you get older, your overall percentage of body fat stays the same, although it is distributed differently as you age.

Your organs age and may malfunction. Your immune system changes, making it harder for your body to fend off or fight disease. And your hearing, eyesight, and other senses (including your sense of balance) all decline to some degree.

Not a pleasant aging scenario? Don't worry: You can take control. There are things you can do to prevent or reverse many of these declines and keep your body at optimal health. A large part of physical health is about self-care and self-initiated preventive health. The other part involves finding a good medical team to support you.

Keep What You've Got—Stay Active

Keeping what you've got is all about prevention. Approximately 82 percent of Americans are not taking the affordable and simple steps to a healthier life, according to a 2008 nationwide survey sponsored by Erickson Health. Staying active is one of the most important steps.

Identify exactly what you want to keep regarding your physical health. The ability to perform daily activities without assistance? Staying free of disease? Avoiding pain and disability? Being active can help in all of these areas. Research shows that even a moderate amount of activity can improve older adults' health, even in the presence of health conditions that may accompany aging. Just walking, which many of us take for granted, has remarkable benefits. Always talk to your doctor before beginning any exercise or activity program.

Stem Cells: Why All the Fuss?

A stem cell is a type of cell that can grow into almost anything. There are primarily two types: those found in adults, and those that come from embryos. Stem cells are not limited to a set number of replications; they can keep photocopying themselves indefinitely. For this reason, stem cells are sometimes referred to as a "fountain of youth." But they need to be biochemically triggered to perform their amazing feats.

The controversy around stem cells lies in the fact that embryonic stem cells are the most versatile for research purposes, but embryos have to be destroyed to perform the research. Obtaining less-versatile stem cells from adults carries minimal health risks to the cell donor.

Scientists are busy studying how to biochemically trigger stem cells to grow for many practical purposes, including regrowing damaged heart muscle and repairing other aging organs and tissues.

Telomerase: A Magic Elixir?

Science says there may be something within cells that helps extend their replication period. This something is called a telomere. A telomere is part of a chromosome (the threadlike packages of genes and DNA contained within your cells).

Telomeres have a nasty habit of shortening every time a cell divides. Once the telomere gets to a certain point, cell replication stops.

A breakthrough discovery (not yet available in your drugstore) called telomerase may help slow down the telomere shortening process. Scientists found that activating telomerase in worms helped them live longer. It's true that humans are a long way from worms, but you may be hearing more about telomerase and longevity research.

Giving Back to the Appalachian Trail

Rob is a seventy-nine-year-old who used to hike the Appalachian Trail regularly. Although he is unable to continue vigorous hiking, he still visits his favorite trail sites for a different purpose—to clean up trash and debris. This monthly activity gives him the opportunity to see favorite sights as well as get some fresh air and moderate exercise.

Helping to clean up the Appalachian Trail has both enjoyment and meaning for Rob—he feels like he is giving back to the trail that has given him so much lifetime pleasure.

If You Think You're Too Old to Exercise . . .

It's never too late to start. Any exercise that promotes strength, balance, stretching of your muscles, and endurance can add years to your life. Some exercises and activities, however, are more age-friendly than others—walking, for instance, whether alone, with a friend, or even with your dog. Playing with grandchildren is another example. And water activities (swimming or water aerobics) don't stress joints and are particularly good for people with arthritis or muscle stiffness. Research supports the heart-healthy benefits of gardening—at least thirty minutes of gardening qualifies as a low-intensity fitness routine as defined by the Centers for Disease Control and Prevention. Gardening has also been shown to help beat depression.

There are even fitness centers that have equipment specifically designed for older adults, with features like easy-to-read display panels, wide, comfortable seats, slow starting speeds, and even low-resistance strength training equipment that uses hydraulics instead of heavy weights. Some fitness centers also offer age-friendly classes like chair aerobics or tai chi. The SilverSneakers program gives you an easy way to find age-friendly gyms; go to www.silversneakers.com for more information.

Find Something You Enjoy

Take inventory: What do you do to stay active on a daily basis? You don't have to start a rigorous, structured exercise program. Buy a pedometer at any sporting-goods store to measure how many walking steps you take each day and aim for ten thousand. There are many ways to get fit—some are low-tech, such as a daily walk, and some are high-tech like using a fitness center machine or activity-focused video games. (At Erickson communities we've had good success with the Nintendo Wii system, in which you can bowl, play tennis, box, or golf—on teams or individually. Now they even have a fun exercise game called WiiFit.) Try fun and social activities like square dancing or ballroom dancing, or look into community volunteering opportunities that involve physical activity (like park cleanup).

Get motivated.

According to the Federal Interagency Forum on Aging-Related Statistics, there was no significant change in the percentage of older people engaged in physical activity between 1997 and 2006, despite a wealth of knowledge and research that supports the benefits of physical activity. A lack of motivation could be one reason.

Finding an activity you enjoy is the first step to getting motivated. Most people agree that exercise is important to physical health. Many people buy videos or books to get inspired.

Many people start exercising. But some studies show that nearly three out of four people who begin exercising drop out within six months. Most likely these people have lost their initial motivation.

In 2006 a United Kingdom research team set out to find out why people lose their motivation to make healthy changes. They found that people experienced either negative motivation or positive motivation. People who tended to have negative motivation (motivation driven by guilt, fear, or regret) tended to slip back into their old unhealthy ways. On the other hand, people who had positive motivation ("I will have more energy to play with my grandkids if I walk every day") tended to stick with their chosen program.

Remember, small investments of time and energy in exercise have positive results. In 2007, the National Health and Medical Research Council, Colonial Foundation, and

Shepherd Foundation conducted a study on walking that found walking is not only good for the heart but good for the knees because it reduces the risk of bone marrow problems and improves the cartilage in the knee.

What motivates you? If it's negative thinking, identify some personal, positive reasons to keep going. Or at least commit to a temporary goal: Some research suggests that doing *something* (especially an activity or exercise) every day for ninety days helps to ingrain it as a habit, and you'll be less likely to abandon your chosen program. Do not start with a rigorous exercise program; rather, build up your exercise and always check with your doctor.

Find a partner.
Having an exercise partner helps you stay accountable to yourself for whatever fitness activity you choose. And it makes it more fun.

Kathy, age eighty-one, would never describe herself as a "happy exerciser." The only activity she really enjoyed was tennis, which she played three times a week soon after she retired. After being injured in a fall, however, she gave it up despite fully recovering from her injuries. Going to a fitness center seemed like too much effort. She thought about walking, but she knew she wouldn't commit to a regular schedule.

During lunch one day, Kathy learned that her new friend Margaret (age eighty-two) also had good intentions about a regular walking schedule but never followed through. They agreed to set up a schedule and stick to it—meeting in the mornings at nine for a half-hour walk.

Seven years later, they're still walking. Although their schedules vary at times because of prior commitments or an occasional illness, their commitment to each other keeps them going. Along with the physical benefits of walking, they also share their problems and joys about their children and grandchildren, and other interesting topics. As Kathy says, "Walking with a partner is not only good for the physical heart, but also for the emotional heart."

Join an exercise group.
Joining an exercise or walking group is a good idea if you need a lot of flexibility and want to meet people. It's a good way to begin an activity program, but it may not be the best way to continue one for the long haul.

The difference between a walking group and a single walking partner is accountability. If you simply don't feel like walking on a particular occasion, you know that the walking group will still walk. If, on the other hand, you usually walk with one partner and don't feel like going one day, your partner may encourage you to go anyway because he/she doesn't want to walk alone!

The people who tend to show up regularly for exercise or walking groups are those who have developed a personal connection with one or two others in the group. So if you join a group, get to know other members.

Keeping What You've Got from the Inside Out: Eating Right

Everyone knows you have to eat well to stay healthy. But with all of the changing information out there, how do you decide which foods to choose? How do you know how much fat, carbohydrates, and protein are in each food and how much is healthy for you? Although individual health needs differ, and you should always check with your doctor or a nutritionist before making any major dietary changes, almost everyone can benefit from these seven features of a healthful diet.

1. Antioxidants. Antioxidants can protect your cells from damage caused by certain chemical reactions (called oxidative processes) in your body. Oxidative processes generate substances called free radicals that may play a role in heart disease, cancer, and some other diseases, like age-related macular degeneration—a disease characterized by a gradual loss of central vision.

Some examples of antioxidants are vitamins A, C, and E, beta-carotene, lutein, lycopene, polyphenols, and selenium. Good dietary sources of these antioxidants include:

- vitamin A and beta-carotene: carrots, spinach, cantaloupe, winter squash

- vitamin C: citrus fruits, broccoli, strawberries, tomatoes

- vitamin E: nuts, seeds, vegetable oils, wheat germ

- lutein: grapes, kiwifruit, spinach, squash

- lycopene: tomato products, watermelon, pink grapefruit

- polyphenols: all teas, especially green tea

- selenium: fish and shellfish, whole grains, eggs

2. Flavonoids. These compounds seem to have various beneficial anti-aging effects on your body. They can boost your immune system and act as antioxidants. Flavonoids are found in blueberries and other dark berries, tea (especially green tea), red grape skins and red wine, red beans, and dark chocolate.

3. Omega-3 fatty acids. Omega-3 fatty acids are considered "essential" fatty acids because they can't be manufactured by the body and so must be obtained from food or supplements. They may have some very real health benefits—studies suggest that high cholesterol and high blood pressure may be reduced with a diet rich in omega-3s, and they may have benefits for the aging brain. Omega-3s are found primarily in cold-water fish or fatty fish like salmon and tuna. They are also found in some plants, nuts, and oils and are the primary active ingredient in fish oil supplements.

4. Low cholesterol. Cholesterol, a waxy, fatlike substance, occurs naturally in all parts of the body. Your body needs some cholesterol to work properly. But if you have too much in your blood, it can stick to the walls of your arteries. This is called plaque. Plaque can narrow your arteries or even block them, leading to heart disease, strokes, and possibly other conditions like Alzheimer's disease. Cholesterol in food only comes from animal-based products, and about one-third to one-fourth of your total blood cholesterol comes from what you eat. Reduce your cholesterol intake by eating only lean meats and low-fat dairy products, and avoid animal-based fats (like lard) found in packaged or prepared foods.

5. Low fat. Some fats are better than others, so make sure the fats in your low-fat foods are healthful ones. Avoid animal-based, saturated, and hydrogenated ("trans") fats because these types of fats contribute to plaque buildup in your arteries. Instead use plant-based unsaturated fats like olive, canola, and sunflower oils. These types of fats don't tend to build up in your arteries, and some research has shown that use of unsaturated fats may help to improve your overall cholesterol profile.

6. Plenty of liquids. Unless you are on a medically imposed fluid restriction, strive for eight (eight-ounce) glasses of fluids (mostly water; avoid caffeine and alcohol) per day, if you are active. Staying well hydrated keeps all of your bodily functions operating at peak efficiency and can help you feel more alert. If you wait until you are thirsty to drink, you've waited too long. By the time your brain sends "thirsty!" signals, you are already dehydrated to some degree so stay ahead of the game. If you are not very active, ask your doctor how many ounces you should strive for.

7. Vitamins. You tend to eat fewer calories as you age and therefore may not get all of the vitamins you need from your daily meals. Depending on your health conditions, age, or sex, you may require additional amounts of a particular vitamin or mineral (postmenopausal women, for example, may need additional calcium and vitamin D) or a multivitamin supplement. Always check with your doctor before starting a multivitamin supplement, and never take a single large dose of any vitamin or mineral without your doctor's consent.

Mother Nature has ensured that your body gets optimal vitamin benefits from food, primarily because of other substances contained in foods that help your body reap a particular vitamin's maximum benefits. Rather than rely on a multivitamin, it's best to get your vitamins by choosing nutrition-packed foods.

8. Carbohydrates. Just like not all fats are bad, not all carbohydrates are good. Carbohydrates are sugars and starches and are part of a complete diet like proteins and fats. Athletes usually consume lots of carbohydrates because of their "energy" or caloric value that is normally burned off by the body during rigorous exercise. Most people do not fit in this category. And if you are a diabetic, you need to monitor the amount of carbohydrates you consume as this can directly impact your blood glucose (sugar) level. Carbohydrates are found in most foods, including vegetables. Potatoes are about 17 percent carbohydrates, while lima beans are about 64 percent carbohydrates. A healthy diet includes moderation in carbohydrates.

Spotlight on Vitamin D

Vitamin D may be the single most important vitamin you're not getting enough of. We know that vitamin D helps you form and maintain strong bones by promoting the absorption of calcium, and more research is showing that vitamin D has a positive effect on your immune system and muscles, and may help reduce breast and colon cancer risk.

Some preliminary research has shown that low levels of vitamin D may be associated with premature death from a variety of causes, including cardiovascular disease.

Vitamin D is measured in international units (IUs), a standard measurement for certain vitamins. The United States Food and Nutrition Board recommended intake is four hundred IUs/day. Some experts, however, think even one thousand to two thousand IUs/per day may be a conservative estimate for older adults, especially women. Getting that much from food is practically impossible, and amounts in multivitamins can vary widely, from fifty IUs to one thousand IUs.

Although the body is designed to make vitamin D when the skin is exposed to sunlight, today's lifestyles,

(continued)

along with skin cancer risks, make it impractical (especially for older adults) to get enough sun to make adequate vitamin D.

Vitamin D is known as a fat-soluble vitamin, which means it's a compound that can be stored in the liver and fatty body tissues. But it doesn't build up in your body the way most people think. Research indicates that it's difficult to reach toxicity levels unless you are taking more than ten thousand IUs/day.

Having low vitamin D levels is not something you can feel. Your doctor can order a simple blood test to determine if you are vitamin D deficient.

Selected Food Sources of Vitamin D

Food/IUs

Salmon, cooked, 3.5 ounces/360

Mackerel, cooked, 3.5 ounces/345

Tuna fish, canned in oil, 3 ounces/200

Sardines, canned in oil, drained, 1.75 ounces/250

Milk, nonfat, reduced fat, and whole, vitamin D-fortified, 1 cup/98

Margarine, fortified, 1 tablespoon/60

Egg, 1 whole (vitamin D is found in yolk)/20

Liver, beef, cooked, 3.5 ounces/15

Cheese, Swiss, 1 ounce/12

Note: Although cod liver oil is high in vitamin D, it is not a good source for older adults because it also contains high levels of vitamin A, which can quickly build up to toxic levels.

A Model for Eating Right

If you stick to a diverse, colorful diet, you're on the right track. Choose foods that are fresh and represent of as many colors as possible (purple eggplant, orange salmon, and green spinach, for example). Following the dietary principles of the much-touted Mediterranean diet is also a good guideline to better nutrition.

There is no one single Mediterranean diet, as several countries border the Mediterranean Sea, but the general principles are a diet high in fresh vegetables, fruits, whole grains, beans, legumes, nuts, and seeds; moderate to high in fish; low in red meat; low to moderate in dairy products; the use of primarily unsaturated fats such as olive oils; and a low intake (one to two glasses per day) of alcohol, mostly in the form of wine.

The Mediterranean diet may reduce your risk of heart disease and other illnesses. Studies have shown that both men and women who consumed Mediterranean diets significantly lowered their risk of heart disease and diabetes compared to similar individuals on low-fat diets.

Pay Attention to Portions

You don't have to eat a lot to have a well-balanced, nutrition-packed diet. If you are concerned about your weight, watch your portion size. In many U.S. restaurants, grocery stores, and even vending machines, portion sizes of both fresh and packaged foods have increased, especially over the last twenty years. Research shows that you tend to eat more when given larger portions.

Serving sizes as listed on most packaged foods are equal to one serving. A serving, however, is not a portion. A serving is the recommended amount of food from that particular food group. For example, a half cup of cooked rice or pasta is considered one serving of grains. Three ounces of meat (the size of a deck of cards) is considered one serving. Visit the United States Department of Agriculture's MyPyramid. gov to customize your recommended daily servings for each food category.

Is Stress Making (or Keeping) You Fat?

Extra fat tends to accumulate at your waist as you age. If you notice an increase, stress may be a culprit, driving you to make unhealthy food choices. Recent research found that rats under stress tended to eat junk foods rather than healthful foods. Examine your taste preferences, cost constraints, or convenience-motivated habits. These lifestyle choices can also drive you to eat junk foods.

Who Is Considered Obese?

The Centers for Disease Control and Prevention (CDC) defines obesity as having a body mass index (BMI) of 30 or

---

High-Risk Fat: Measure Your Waist

Several studies have shown that an easy and simple way to monitor your health is to measure your waist. Many previous studies have focused on body weight in relation to height (body mass index, or BMI) as an ideal health indicator, but newer information lends more credence to waist size as a way to determine, for both sexes, who is at a higher overall health risk—particularly for conditions such as high blood pressure, diabetes, and elevated cholesterol. Think of excess waist fat as "high-risk" fat.

How to measure: Using a tape measure, find the midway point between the bottom of your ribcage and the top of your pelvic bones. Stand up straight

---

greater. BMI is calculated using your height and weight and provides a reasonable indicator of weight *categories* that may lead to health problems. Obesity is a major risk factor for heart disease, certain cancers, and type 2 diabetes.

The CDC reports that adults ages forty to fifty-nine have the highest prevalence of obesity compared to other groups. Approximately 40 percent of men in this age group were obese, compared to 32 percent of men sixty and older. Among women, 41 percent of those ages forty to fifty-nine were obese compared to 30.5 percent of women ages sixty-five and older.

All individuals vary, and there are plenty of overweight people who are vigorously healthy, as well as normal weight individuals with a large number of health problems; so you should always consult your doctor before deciding to undergo a weight-loss regimen or making any major nutrition changes.

(don't suck in your stomach!) and measure your waist circumference at that halfway point.

Everyone will have variations depending upon height and body type, but the International Diabetes Federation recommends the following guidelines:

Waist measurement upper limits by primary race and sex

Caucasian, African, or Middle Eastern descent
Males, 37 inches   Females, 31.5 inches
Latino or Asian descent
Males, 35.5 inches   Females, 31.5 inches

These measurements are guidelines only. Check with your doctor if you think you are at an increased risk of health problems.

How to Incorporate Inexpensive and Healthy Meals into Your Routine

Erickson's executive chefs talk to our residents daily and know how difficult it can be to choose nutritious foods regularly, especially if you are on a budget. Here are some of their suggestions for saving money, eating healthfully, and buying foods economically.

Read grocery ads first and then plan your weekly menu accordingly. Grocery stores often put their freshest in-season produce on sale. Fresh produce has a high nutritional value. Also look for sales on lean meats, fish, and whole grain pastas, breads, or rice.

Planning your menu with grocery sale items in mind before you shop helps you avoid buying higher-priced convenience items that may not be as healthful. Having a set grocery list for your weekly menu plan also helps you avoid the bombardment of in-store advertising often featuring higher-priced, non-nutritious choices.

Shop at farmers' markets or ethnic markets. Both farmers' markets and ethnic groceries tend to have fresh produce at low prices. Asian groceries, in particular, tend to have fresh fish at reasonable prices.

Keep meals simple with three or four main ingredients. Meals made with fewer ingredients tend to be the most healthful and economical. Choose from the freshest ingredients and other items that are on sale that week.

Use your leftovers. Think salads, soups, sandwiches. With leftover pork, make barbecued pork sandwiches. Make chicken salad from leftover chicken. If you have a lot of vegetables, pasta, or rice, make a quick soup by adding a can of tomato or French onion soup and some spices. Use leftover vegetables to make salads or side dishes.

Eat breakfast foods for dinner once a week. This is also a great way to use leftovers. Incorporate leftover meats and vegetables into an egg white omelet or quiche. Serve with whole wheat toast. Breakfast-type foods also tend to be economical—try corn pancakes with diced ham or whole wheat and turkey bacon waffles.

Try a meatless entrée once a week. Going meatless is a big cost saver. Try a vegetable stir-fry with brown rice, a vegetable lasagna made with whole wheat noodles, or bean and cheese burritos using whole wheat tortillas.

Buy in bulk. Whether you buy in bulk at your regular grocery or at wholesale stores, buying in bulk is a great value, especially for rice, pastas, and beans, even though some grain prices have risen in the past few years. Prepackaged and seasoned varieties of these products tend to cost two or even three times as much, and tend to be high in sodium. Buying in bulk also means you can cook in advance, use custom seasonings, and use the prepared products as bases for meals throughout the week. Don't forget meat—buying meat in bulk packages can save you money. Use a food-saver device to portion out meats for freezing.

Dine out in the early part of the week. More restaurants use incentives and specials to attract customers on Mondays, Tuesdays, and Wednesdays. Very often you'll find half-price entrees or even two-for-one specials on these days. Check your local paper or flyers for early week specials. The same holds true for dining earlier in the day; arriving before four or five gets you special prices in many cases.

Simple Meal Ideas from Our Chefs

For breakfast, have oatmeal with apple slices and milk, or an egg white omelet with spinach, cheese, and some whole wheat toast. For lunch, make chicken salad with grapes on whole wheat bread or rolls, or a tuna salad–stuffed tomato. For dinner, try whole wheat pasta, a small amount of canned sauce, and low-fat ground beef or chicken for a quick and healthful spaghetti with meat sauce. Or roast a pork loin with potatoes and carrots in one pan and coat with a store-bought pesto sauce before serving. Have a chicken with zucchini, tomatoes, and potatoes coated with olive oil and fresh herbs—all roasted in one pan. Add a salad and whole wheat rolls. For lunch or dinner you can always serve pizza made with premade dough and topped with fresh and healthful ingredients like chicken, shrimp, broccoli, spinach, mushrooms, parmesan, or low-fat mozzarella cheese.

All of these suggestions are great for guests or grandchildren, and if it's just one or two of you, you'll have plenty of leftovers. Below we've included some of our most popular recipes in case you'd like to try a few of them yourself.

Recipes from Our Chefs
Following are some delicious and healthful recipes from our chefs in Erickson communities nationwide.

GAZPACHO: SERVES 10

2 cans tomato juice (approximately 46 ounces)
2 cups water
1 cucumber, peeled, seeded, and finely diced
1 tablespoon fresh garlic, minced
¼ cup each (chopped) red bell pepper, green pepper, onion, zucchini, and carrots
1 tablespoon sugar
3 tablespoons red wine vinegar
1 tablespoon olive oil
½ teaspoon cayenne pepper
Dash of hot sauce
1 tablespoon chives
2 tablespoons fresh cilantro, chopped
2 tablespoons scallions, chopped

(continued)

46

Mix together tomato juice, water, diced cucumber, and minced garlic in a large bowl. Put red and green peppers, onion, zucchini, and carrots into a food processor and pulse twice. Add to tomato mixture. Add remaining ingredients, stir, and chill well before serving.

WHITE BEAN SOUP WITH ESCAROLE, SWEET POTATOES, AND SAUSAGE: SERVES 6–8

1 cup dried white cannellini beans
½ cup dry white table wine
8 cups low-sodium chicken broth
1/3 cup Spanish onion, diced
½ teaspoon garlic, minced
½ cup crushed tomatoes
2 large sweet potatoes, peeled and cut into 1-inch cubes
1/3 cup carrots, diced
1 pound mild Italian turkey sausage, cooked and cut into ¼-inch pieces
One head escarole lettuce, washed and chopped
2 bay leaves
Salt and pepper to taste
Olive oil, for drizzling
Parmesan cheese

Place white beans in a quart of cold water and refrigerate uncovered overnight. The next day, drain and rinse beans and place them in a large stock pot with white wine, chicken broth, onion, garlic, and crushed tomatoes. Bring to a boil, lower heat, and allow to simmer until beans are almost cooked through—about 20 to 25 minutes.

(continued)

Add sweet potatoes and carrots, cooking until beans are soft yet firm and sweet potatoes are tender—about another 20 minutes.

Remove from heat. Carefully ladle about 2½ cups of broth and the bean-potato mixture into a blender. Puree until smooth.

Add blended mixture back into the stock pot along with sausage, escarole, and bay leaves. Mix soup to incorporate the puree. Add salt and pepper to taste. Heat on low for another 10 or 15 minutes. Remove bay leaves. Serve drizzled with olive oil and topped with Parmesan cheese.

THE POWER WRAP: SERVES 1

1 10-inch spinach-flavored tortilla
½ teaspoon horseradish
3 tablespoons light mayonnaise
⅓ cup grated Gouda cheese
4 ounces turkey breast, sliced thin
3 slices tomato
1 large lettuce leaf

Place tortilla on cutting surface. Mix horseradish and mayonnaise and spread evenly over tortilla, stopping about ½ inch from edge. Sprinkle cheese over this.

Top with turkey breast, tomato, and lettuce. Taking the edge closest to you, fold the edge about 1 inch over the filling and roll halfway. Then fold in the sides to the right and left toward the center—make it nice and tight. Continue to roll; when completed it should look like a giant egg roll. Cut in half and serve with fresh fruit.

BUTTERMILK CHICKEN: SERVES 4

4 boneless, skinless chicken breasts (approximately one pound)
2 cups buttermilk
2 cups all-purpose flour
1 cup bread crumbs
½ teaspoon lemon pepper seasoning
½ teaspoon tarragon
½ cup melted margarine
½ teaspoon paprika
Salt and pepper to taste
1 cup mustard salad dressing
1 teaspoon chopped chives

Marinate chicken in buttermilk in a covered, nonmetallic container and refrigerate for at least two hours. Combine dry ingredients (flour, bread crumbs, lemon pepper seasoning, tarragon, paprika, salt and pepper).

Discard marinade and dredge chicken in flour mixture, coating well. Place chicken on greased baking pan and drizzle with margarine. Bake at 375° for approximately 40 to 45 minutes or until internal temperature reaches 165°. Drizzle chicken with mustard dressing and top with chives.

HONEY DIJON SALMON: SERVES 4

½ cup honey
2 tablespoons Dijon mustard
1½ tablespoons melted butter or margarine
2 teaspoons Worcestershire sauce
1 tablespoon cornstarch
1/8 teaspoon white pepper
1 pound fresh asparagus
4 salmon steaks
1/3 cup chopped walnuts

Preheat oven to 450°. Prepare 4 (12 x 18-inch) sheets of aluminum foil and set aside. Blend honey, mustard, butter, Worcestershire sauce, cornstarch, and pepper. Set aside.

Center ¼ of asparagus on each sheet of foil. Top with salmon steaks. Drizzle each salmon steak with ¼ of honey-mustard sauce and top with chopped walnuts.

Bring up the sides of each foil sheet to meet in the middle. Double fold the top and ends to seal packets, leaving a pocket of air for heat circulation inside. Place packets on baking sheet and bake 17 to 23 minutes. Carefully pierce packets to release steam before opening.

SPRING VEGETABLES WITH LEMON AND SHALLOTS: SERVES 6

3 pounds fresh fava beans, shelled
2 tablespoons olive oil, divided
1 tablespoon unsalted butter or margarine, divided
4 shallots, finely sliced
1 pound sugar snap peas, trimmed
1 pound asparagus, trimmed and cut diagonally into
    ½-inch pieces
2 (3-inch) strips lemon zest, julienned
2 teaspoons fresh lemon juice
Salt and pepper to taste

To prepare fava beans, blanch for 1 minute, then cool and remove outer skins. (One pound frozen Fordhook lima beans may be substituted for fava beans but also should be blanched and set aside.)

In a large skillet, heat 1 tablespoon oil and ½ tablespoon butter over moderately high heat. Sauté shallots, stirring until tender, about 2 minutes. With a slotted spoon transfer shallots to a bowl. Sauté snap peas in the remaining oil, stirring occasionally until crisp yet tender.

In another skillet, heat remaining oil and butter over moderately high heat. Sauté asparagus, stirring occasionally until crisp yet tender. Add fava or lima beans and sauté for about 2 minutes.

Add zest, lemon juice, snap peas, shallots, and salt and pepper to taste, and sauté until just heated through.

APPLE COBBLER WITH STREUSEL TOPPING:
SERVES 4

5 cups tart apples, peeled and sliced
¼ cup sugar
2 tablespoons all-purpose flour
½ teaspoon cinnamon
¼ teaspoon salt
1 teaspoon vanilla extract
¼ cup water
1 tablespoon butter or margarine, softened
Topping:
½ cup all-purpose flour, sifted
½ cup sugar
¼ teaspoon salt
2 tablespoons butter or margarine, softened

In a medium bowl, mix together apples, sugar, flour, cinnamon, salt, vanilla, and water. Spoon apple mixture into a lightly greased 9-inch square baking pan. Dot apples with 1 tablespoon butter or margarine.

Combine all topping ingredients and mix together until crumbs form. Sprinkle topping over apple mixture. Bake 35 to 40 minutes at 375° or until apples are tender. Serve with vanilla frozen yogurt or ice cream.

STRAWBERRY SHORTCAKE: SERVES 5

½ cup + 1 tablespoon all-purpose flour
2¼ teaspoons baking powder
5 teaspoons solid shortening
¼ cup + 5 teaspoons milk
1¼ teaspoons sugar
$3/8$ teaspoon salt
1 small egg, beaten
2½ cups sliced strawberries
Whipped topping for garnish

Preheat oven to 450°. Combine flour and baking powder. Cut shortening into flour until crumbly.

Combine milk, sugar, salt, and egg. Mix well and add to flour mixture. Mix lightly.

Pat out dough on floured board to 1-inch thickness. Fold all four corners into center. Repeat folding two or three more times. Roll out dough to 1-inch thickness. Cut with a 2-inch cutter and place on ungreased baking sheet. Bake for 12 to 15 minutes.

Split biscuits in half. Place bottom half in sherbet dish and spoon ¼ cup strawberries over top. Place top of biscuit on strawberries. Ladle another ¼ cup strawberries over top. Top each shortcake with a dollop of whipped topping. Serve immediately.

Eating Better Than Ever Despite Diabetes

Ian is fifty-five years old and has always taken pride in his active lifestyle. He runs every day and also enjoys golfing on a regular basis. Although type 2 diabetes runs in his family, Ian always thought that because he was so fit, he stood little chance of getting the disease. So Ian was quite surprised when he was recently diagnosed.

Treatment-wise, Ian's doctor recommended medication, blood glucose monitoring, continued activity, and dietary changes. Ian always thought that his diet was fairly well balanced until he examined it carefully. He realized that he ate quite a bit of refined sugar in the form of cookies and sweetened drinks. His diet was also heavy in other carbohydrates, like potatoes, white rice, and bread.

Ian changed his diet. He added more vegetables and whole grains. He chose lean meats and used sugar substitutes to satisfy his sweet tooth. Ian found that his new eating plan had a number of benefits. Because he chose high-fiber, nutrition-packed foods, he ate less and felt more satisfied after meals. His grocery bills decreased because he planned his meals every week. Best of all, Ian's blood glucose readings greatly improved.

Secret #4: Find Your Team

If you own (or have ever owned) a car, think of how you take care of it. If it needs gas, you fill up at the gas station. If the brakes don't feel right or you need an oil change, you take it to a mechanic. If it needs tires, you go to a tire store.

Some people treat their health care in the same fragmented way. If they have foot pain, they seek out a podiatrist. If they're experiencing vision changes, they go to an eye doctor. And they see yet another doctor for an annual physical. Yet other people have prescriptions filled at more than one pharmacy, and some choose a walk-in clinic if they have a cold, rather than call their regular doctor.

When it comes to your car, if you're really lucky you have one trusted mechanic who can do all of your services for you, and if not, can refer you to another trusted source for outlying problems. When it comes to your health, you're even more fortunate if you have one doctor who can coordinate all of your health care needs.

At Erickson, we believe in the "medical home" model of health care. A medical home is not a building or a hospital, but rather a team approach to health care. It starts with a trusted primary physician with whom you form a partnership. Your doctor and office staff coordinate your care with you, your specialists, your family, and other resources so that you receive all the needed services to maximize your health and independence.

A 2008 University of Utah study showed that team-based care improved quality of life and lowered care costs for older adults, especially for people with chronic health conditions. Coordinated, integrated care is of high value because it results in better outcomes at lower cost to you. It means having fewer tests, fewer doctor visits, and perhaps even fewer surgeries and hospitalizations. It reduces medication errors and side effects because you have one primary care doctor managing your medicines rather than four or five specialists who typically do not know what the others are prescribing. In a 2003 survey released by the Commonwealth Fund, one in three American adults reported that in the past two years, their doctors had ordered an already-performed test or recommended unnecessary treatment. The survey also revealed that many respondents were frustrated with the way they currently receive health care. Almost half of the people surveyed experienced poorly coordinated medical care, including not being informed about test results or having to call repeatedly to get them, as well as poor communication between doctors and nurses and primary doctors and specialists.

The Medical Home Concept

The term "medical home" might seem like a technical term, but it's actually a simple concept. Your doctor coordinates your medical care. This care coordination prevents unnecessary treatments and may help you avoid potential complications related to your health, thus keeping you as active and independent as possible. The American Academy of Pediatrics introduced the medical home concept in 1967. The term in those days referred mainly to the concept of archiving a child's medical record in one central location. Since then, the concept has expanded and the following principles of a patient-centered medical "home" were jointly developed by the American Academy of Family Physicians, the American Academy of Pediatrics, American College of Physicians, and the American Osteopathic Association.

Personal physician: Each patient has an ongoing relationship with a personal physician trained to provide first contact and continuous and comprehensive care.

Physician-directed medical practice: The personal physician leads a team of individuals at the practice level who collectively take responsibility for the continued care of patients.

Whole-person orientation: The personal physician is responsible for fulfilling all the patient's health care needs or taking responsibility for appropriately arranging care with other qualified professionals. This includes preventive services, acute care, chronic care, and end-of-life care.

Coordinated and/or integrated care: This coordination/integration includes care across all elements of the health care system (subspecialty care, hospitals, home health agencies, nursing homes) and the patient's community (family, public, and private community-based services). Care is facilitated by information technology and other means to assure that patients get the indicated care when and where they need and want it in a culturally and linguistically appropriate manner.

Quality and safety: This includes features such as patient advocacy, physician accountability, the use of information technology, a voluntary review process to ensure adherence to medical home model concepts, and quality improvement programs.

Enhanced access to care: This includes making care available through systems such as open scheduling, expanded hours, and new options for communication among patients, their personal physician, and practice staff.

Payment/added value: A payment structure is devised that appropriately recognizes the added value provided to those who have a patient-centered medical home. This structure protects patients and insurance companies from being charged for extraneous services and helps keep overall health care costs down.

What to look for in your medical home

What can you take away from these principles when searching for your medical home? Chances are you won't see the term "medical home" either in advertisements or in anything printed from a doctor's office. Although the concept has been around for a while, the terminology is not yet in regular use. If you are looking for a medical home, focus on three features.

A personal and caring physician relationship. You want someone who sees you as a whole person, not just a diabetic, arthritis sufferer, heart patient, and so on. Does your doctor ask you about all aspects of your life or just focus on your health problems? Does he/she make sure you understand what you need to do to take care of yourself? Do you have time to ask all of your questions? Do you have access to a doctor on nights and weekends?

Doctor-directed care coordination. Is there someone to help coordinate your care both before and after your appointments? Look for a well-trained staff who make your follow-up appointments and referrals to laboratories, radiology offices, or other specialists easy for you. Does your doctor have relationships with specialists and community resources? Can he or she help you with second opinions and offer suggestions or alternatives to treatments suggested by other doctors? Your doctor should keep track of your care and communicate with your specialists and with you.

Electronic medical records. This can be difficult to find, because few (estimates range anywhere from 5 percent to 18 percent) doctors' offices use a fully integrated electronic medical records system. A fully integrated system allows your doctor to easily communicate your safely stored medical information in real time to specialists, emergency rooms, pharmacies, and so on. If you can't find a doctor that has electronic medical records, look for signs of efficiency where your medical records are concerned. Can staff access your records quickly if you need them for a referral? Do they return your phone calls quickly? Is it easy to make appointments? Are your prescription requests handled quickly and accurately?

People who seek their health care through a medical home get better quality care and are more satisfied with the care they receive. Their experiences don't reflect assembly-line care because their doctors and staff know them well. They've found their team.

What NOT to Look For in Your Medical Home: The Story of Bubba's Shingles

Bubba walked into a doctor's office. The receptionist asked him what he had. Bubba said, "Shingles." The receptionist took his personal and medical insurance information and asked him to have a seat.

Fifteen minutes later, a nurse's aide asked Bubba what he had. Bubba said, "Shingles." The nurse's aide checked his height, weight, and medical history and asked Bubba to wait in the examining room.

Thirty minutes later, a nurse came into the room and asked Bubba what he had. Bubba said, "Shingles." The nurse checked his temperature and blood pressure and took a blood sample and told him to take off his clothes and wait for the doctor.

One hour later, the doctor came in, found Bubba sitting in the nude, and asked him what he had. Bubba said, "Shingles." The doctor asked, "Where?"

Bubba said, "Outside on the truck. Where do you want me to unload 'em?"

A Medical Home's Response to an Emergency

Elaine was skiing with her husband when she had an accident that sent her to the emergency room.

Because Elaine and her husband had a personal relationship with their physician, Dr. Abin, they called her right away about what had just happened, even though it was Saturday. Dr. Abin accessed Elaine's medical records from her home computer and was able to discuss a treatment plan over the phone with the emergency room physician, including the appropriate medications, lab tests, and discharge plans for Elaine.

Once Elaine was home, Dr. Abin called to check on Elaine's progress and discuss any questions that Elaine or her husband had. As a result Elaine did not have any medication or treatment complications at the hospital and enjoyed a speedy recovery. The following winter, Elaine was back on the ski slopes in top form.

Your Check-ups and Screenings

To keep yourself healthy, you need to have regular check-ups and other recommended screenings. This is part of preventive care. Although some experts disagree about the frequency of regular check-ups, we think that seeing your doctor at least once a year is a good idea—if nothing else to maintain an open relationship with him/her, do a medication review, or answer any questions you might have.

The following chart lists some key screenings for adults. Depending on your family or personal health history, your doctor may recommend a different frequency or additional tests.

Recommended Preventive Health Screenings

	Age 20–40	Age 40–50	Age 50-plus
Routine physical	as needed	as needed	1-2 times/ year
Eye exam	every 2–3 years	every 1–2 years	every year
Blood pressure	every 2 years	every 2 years	every year
Cholesterol	every 5 years	every 5 years	every 5 years
Blood sugar	–	at age 45	every 3 years
Fecal occult blood	–	–	every year
Colonoscopy	–	–	every 3-5 years
Rectal exam	–	–	every year
For men:			
Prostate-specific antigen	–	–	every year until age 75
For women:			
Pap smear	every year	every year	every year until age 70
Do-it-yourself breast exam	monthly	monthly	monthly
Office breast exam	every 3 years	every year	every year
Mammogram	–	every year	every year

Paying for Preventive Care

As evidence mounts about the cost-effectiveness of preventing diseases like the flu, heart disease, and diabetes, Medicare and other insurances are increasingly paying for health screenings and immunizations. Despite this increase in coverage, some surveys show that less than 10 percent of Medicare recipients are getting all of their recommended screenings. Check your Medicare or other insurance benefits. What wasn't covered last year may be covered now.

Empower Yourself and Your Team with Knowledge

A 2008 survey sponsored by Erickson Health shows that a majority of American voters are knowledgeable about some aspects of preventive self-care, such as nutrition and exercise, but many do not recognize the value of preventive screenings. Other research indicates that many Americans are not as knowledgeable as they should be about their own health conditions (such as not knowing the symptoms of a heart attack or stroke) or that they are not taking the right preventive steps toward better health.

Our survey also revealed that while most voters rely on their families for information about preventive health care, voters age sixty-five and older tend to rely on medical professionals and health insurance companies. The majority of your health care information should be obtained from your doctor. But some studies have shown that people, no matter what their age, tend to forget 40 percent to 80 percent of the information their doctors told them by the time they leave the office.

Your Health Literacy

According to the Federal Interagency Forum on Aging-Related Statistics, health literacy is the degree to which people have the capacity to obtain, process, and understand basic health information and services needed to make appropriate health decisions. Adhering to prescription instructions, filling out a patient information form, or giving informed consent are specific tasks that require more than just an adequate level of basic literacy—they require an adequate level of health literacy.

Older adults are proportionately more likely than any other age group to have below average health literacy. Almost 39 percent of people age seventy-five and over have a health literacy level of below average compared with 23 percent of people ages sixty-five to seventy-four and 13 percent of people ages fifty to sixty-four.

More doctors' offices are providing written health information in easy-to-understand forms. Augment your health literacy by asking for written educational information about your health conditions and medications. Communication is important, and some simple directions can be hard to interpret. For example, a doctor may tell you to take a medication three times a day. Does that mean every eight hours? Or is it three times a day during the daytime only? What if you're two hours late taking it? These are important questions that need to be clarified.

Keep your own medical records.

Be knowledgeable about your health and your preventive care, and have a way to communicate your knowledge to your health providers. If you are lucky, your doctor uses electronic medical records. With such a system, you can get a printout or maybe even access portions of your record online to review or print. Ultimately, however, it's up to you

Information to Include
in Your Personal Medical Record

❑ Your personal information: name, address, phone number(s), birth date

❑ Contact information: who to notify in case of emergency, or caregiver name, phone number, and relationship to you

❑ All doctors' names and phone numbers, including your primary doctor and any specialists

❑ Information about any advance directives (living will or medical power of attorney) you may have

❑ Allergies: medications and environmental

❑ Medications: names, dosages, frequency, reason for taking, pharmacy name and phone number (include herbal supplements and vitamins/minerals)

❑ Chronic health conditions (high blood pressure, diabetes, arthritis, etc.)

❑ Major illnesses and injuries and dates of occurrence (cancer, infections, broken bones or other trauma)

❑ Hospitalizations: include emergency room visits/dates/reasons (include major surgeries and dates)

❑ Family history: major diseases and causes of death for family members

❑ Your immunization records

❑ Any current laboratory, health screening, or radiology results

❑ Assistive devices that you use: pacemaker, glasses, hearing aids, cane, walker

to keep your records updated. You can help by formulating your own record and keeping it current. Give updated copies to your doctor and family members or friends who may need it. Take your record with you to medical appointments. Ask for a copy of your records to review for accuracy. Not only can incorrect information lead to medical errors, it could affect your insurability and the price of your premiums.

What You Need to Know about Advance Directives

Advance directives are legal documents that allow you to communicate decisions about your medical care if you lose your decision-making abilities because of an accident or serious illness. These papers are an important part of your medical record.

There are different types of advance directives, and laws pertaining to them vary by state. Common advance directive documents are living wills and durable powers of attorney for health care. Often these two documents can be found on one form.

A living will describes the kind of medical or life-sustaining treatments you would want if you were seriously or terminally ill. It is also known as a directive to physicians, health care declarations, or medical directives.

A living will is limited however, and can't cover all of the bases. You need someone who can make decisions about unexpected medical dilemmas that might arise. That's the function of the durable power of attorney for health care, which names your health care proxy or agent. A durable power of attorney for health care is also known as a medical power of attorney or health

(continued)

---

care power of attorney. Don't confuse it with a traditional or financial power of attorney.

You can obtain forms for advance directives from your health care provider, health department, or lawyer, or online from your state's Web site. To see if an advance directive for your state is available online, Google the name of your state, "medical society" or "bar association," and "advance directive." A good resource from the American Bar Association can also be found at http://abanet.org/aging/toolkit.

Important Points to Remember When Writing Your Advance Directives:

- Have a discussion with your chosen health care agent (family or power of attorney) so he/she fully understands your wishes.

- Keep up-to-date about new life-sustaining measures and technologies.

- Know your state's laws and regulations—especially witnessing and notarizing requirements.

- Keep your original signed documents in an easily accessible place.

- Give your doctor, proxy, and any other necessary people copies of your documents.

- Update/revise your documents every five years or as necessary for medical or other life changes.

Get Back What You Can

As we talked about earlier in this chapter, there are inevitable losses that come with aging, but there are also ways to get back some of what you've lost. In this section, we'll focus on the strategies with the biggest payoffs.

Practice Good Nutrition

If you follow the guidelines in the previous section about nutrition, you will be in better shape to start feeling younger. Following a good diet may help repair some aging damage. It is well documented that a diet low in fat and rich in whole grains can lower your cholesterol. Research is ongoing about the use of fats like olive oils, which may help reverse damage to your blood vessels. And there is emerging research about antioxidants' and omega-3 fatty acids' benefits to many areas of your body, including your eye health. That means eating fish such as salmon every week and drinking green tea (among other things discussed previously in this chapter).

Quit Smoking

Quitting now can help you return to better health. Even if you only smoke three or four cigarettes a day, it can take ten years for your lungs to return to normal, and five years for your liver to return to normal after you've quit. The body has remarkable healing powers. Even if you have smoked for thirty years, you can reduce your risk of heart disease to that of a nonsmoker within five to ten years after stopping.

Quitting can also save you money—not only because cigarettes are increasingly expensive, but because many life insurance companies offer much lower rates to nonsmokers. Even some health insurance plans are starting to offer lower rates and other incentives for nonsmokers.

The bad news about smoking

Facts about older adults and smoking:

- In 2005, 18.7 million Americans over age forty-five smoked (including 9 percent of Americans over age sixty-five), accounting for over 41 percent of all adult smokers.

- Smoking is responsible for 90 percent of lung cancer deaths, 80 percent to 90 percent of deaths from chronic obstructive pulmonary disease (COPD—emphysema and bronchitis), 21 percent of heart disease deaths, and 18 percent of deaths from stroke. All of these health conditions are leading causes of illness and death in people over age fifty.

- Men sixty-five years of age and older who smoke are twice as likely to die from a stroke, and women smokers are one and a half times as likely to die from a stroke than their nonsmoking counterparts age sixty-five and older.

- Cigarette smokers are more than twice as likely as nonsmokers to develop dementia, including Alzheimer's disease.

- Smokers have two to three times the risk of developing cataracts as nonsmokers. Cataracts are opacities of the eye lens that are a major cause of vision loss in older adults.

- Smoking reduces your normal life expectancy by an average of thirteen to fifteen years—thereby eliminating precious retirement years.

In short, you will almost certainly suffer negative health effects if you continue to smoke.

The Good News about Quitting Smoking

You've heard the bad news about smoking, but getting back what you can will go a long way if you quit today. Quitting smoking carries a big payoff for a healthier aging process.

If you quit today . . .

After twenty minutes: Blood pressure and heart rate decrease.

Eight hours: Blood levels of oxygen and carbon dioxide normalize.

One day: Your risk of heart attack begins to decrease.

Two days: Airway starts clearing and your senses of smell and taste improve.

Two weeks to three months: Walking and other activities become easier because your circulation and breathing improve.

One to nine months: You feel more energetic because coughing, sinus congestion, shortness of breath, and fatigue decrease.

One year: Your heart disease risk has been halved.

Five years: Your risks of cancers of the lung, mouth, throat, and esophagus are decreased.

(continued)

Ten years: Your risk of dying from lung cancer is now similar to nonsmokers.

Fifteen years: You are at no more risk of heart disease than if you never smoked.

Getting help to quit

If you still smoke, you're probably running out of places to light up. Many states are enacting legislation that restricts smoking in most public and work areas. Having fewer places to smoke can help motivate you to quit.

It's easier than ever to quit smoking today because of medical advances. Your doctor can help you formulate an individualized plan to stop smoking, as well as prescribe medication or recommend over-the-counter aids that might work best for you.

Enlist the aid of your family and friends, and remember: Even if you don't succeed the first time (most quitters don't), keep trying. Go to Appendix A for more resources for smoking cessation.

Keep Alcohol to a Minimum

If you are like many Americans, you might drink alcohol at least occasionally. For many people, moderate drinking is probably safe. It may even have health benefits, including reducing your risk of certain heart problems. Moderate drinking is considered to be one drink a day for women or anyone over age sixty-five, and two drinks a day for men under sixty-five. One drink is twelve ounces of beer, one and one half ounces of distilled spirits, or five ounces of wine.

Some people should not drink at all, including people on certain medicines and people with some medical conditions. If you have questions about whether it is safe for you to drink, consult your health care provider.

Anything more than moderate drinking can be risky. Binge drinking—drinking five or more drinks at one time— can damage your health and increase your risk for accidents, injuries, and assault. Years of heavy drinking can lead to liver disease, heart disease, cancer, and pancreatitis.

Get Active

Even if you are out of shape or have lost muscle function due to an illness or chronic health condition, engaging in a safe activity program may help you get back some of that lost muscle. Always talk to your doctor before starting any exercise program, especially if your daily functioning has been affected by a lifetime of inactivity or a disease process. Your doctor may recommend physical or occupational therapy to help you get started.

At Erickson communities, our rehabilitation specialists (physical, occupational, and speech therapists) know the fitness principles that work best for older adults. Here are their suggestions for the essential components of any successful activity program:

Always start with a warm-up. Warming up is crucial before beginning any activity, no matter what you choose. Warm up by starting your chosen activity slowly. If you are walking, start slowly and gradually work up to your chosen speed. Warming up is also a period of relaxation in which you can prepare your mind for your upcoming activity.

Include cardiovascular or aerobic exercise in your regimen. Cardiovascular or aerobic activity is brisk physical activity that requires your heart and lungs to work harder to meet the body's increased oxygen demand. Aerobic activity promotes oxygen's circulation through the blood to your vital organs, helps keep your heart in shape, and revs up your metabolism.

Start with as little as five minutes each day of walking, swimming, dancing, or any favorite hobby that is active. Work up to a total of thirty minutes a day for most days of the week. That thirty minutes a day does not have to be all at one time—you can break it into segments if it's more convenient.

Resistance training. We're not talking about strenuous weightlifting. Resistance training is for building muscle and bone strength, and can be especially beneficial if you have osteoporosis or are prone to the disease. You don't have to use fancy machines, either. You can begin with something as simple as a soup can or basic therapeutic elastic bands that are available in many stores. Strengthening your muscles can help combat muscle atrophy and weakness associated with aging, and it may help maintain your metabolism at a more optimal level. Focus on your main muscle groups— your arms, legs, abdomen, and back.

Flexibility training. Flexibility (stretching) exercises help keep you limber by stretching the muscles and tissues that hold your body's structures in place. You can include basic stretching exercises as your warm-up (although stretching can be more effective when done after your muscles are warmed up), or engage in more structured training like yoga classes. Find out from your doctor what kind of flexibility exercises are best for you. Many people require targeted exercises after an illness or injury. And remember: Flexibility training may cause mild discomfort but should never cause pain.

Include a balance component. With aging comes a decreased sense of balance. Many medical conditions, general weakness due to inactivity, changes in your muscles, or other factors can contribute to a lack of balance. Balance training exercises focus on building strength and flexibility while also challenging the sensory systems involved in balance.

If you notice changes in your ability to get in and out of a chair or car, that you are holding on to furniture or the wall more as you're walking, or you're increasingly catching your feet on uneven surfaces and almost falling, you've already developed balance problems. Practicing certain activities can help you prevent a further decline in your sense of balance and may help prevent falls and fractures.

For most balance activities, it's best to see a rehabilitation specialist through a medical center–affiliated rehabilitation department or a wellness center. Balance activities can be simple or they can be more advanced—usually requiring supervision and/or a partner (research supports the benefits of tai chi classes in improving balance for older adults, for example).

Test Your Balance: The Raised-Leg Test

This test was featured in a *New York Times* article by Jane Brody and is based on the work of therapists Marilyn Moffat and Carole B. Lewis. It is adapted from a series of tests recommended by the National Institute on Aging. Before trying this test, make sure you have someone standing by and something sturdy (like a counter or heavy furniture) to steady yourself if necessary.

- Wearing flat, closed shoes, stand up straight with your arms folded across your chest.

- Raise one leg, bending your knee about 45 degrees.

(continued)

- Start a stopwatch and close your eyes.

- Remain on one leg and stop the watch if you uncross your arms, tilt sideways more than 45 degrees, move the leg you're standing on, or touch the floor with your raised leg.

Compare your result with the normal parameters as outlined by Moffat and Lewis:
Age 20 to 49: 24 to 28 seconds
50 to 59: 21 seconds
60 to 69: 10 seconds
70 to 79: 4 seconds
Age 80 and over: Many cannot perform this test.

Test Your Balance: The Sit-to-Stand Test

- Find a sturdy chair with a seat eighteen inches off the floor.

- Sit on the chair with your arms folded.

- Keeping your arms folded, stand up five times as quickly as possible without touching, pushing, or grabbing onto anything.

Evaluating this test is a little tricky depending on the height of the chair, the position of your feet, and the use/availability of armrests.

So be sure that your chair seat is one and a half feet off the floor, your feet are comfortably placed a shoulder's length apart on the floor, and your arms are firmly placed across your chest. It might help to enlist a family member or friend to watch you stand up in this assessment.

Results, as summarized in the journal *Physical Therapy*:

If you stood up quickly and without any trouble at all, then you are in great shape according to this test.

If you stood up fairly quickly but seemed to teeter a little bit or move your feet to gain your balance as you were standing up, then consider asking your doctor to watch you as you do this test.

If you stood up fairly quickly but needed to lean on an armrest, rocked your body back to gain momentum to stand up, or had to put something on the seat to make it higher, then again consider discussing this with your doctor.

If you could not stand up at all or without pushing yourself up with your arms, then discuss your options with your doctor.

Simple Balance Activities

- Stand up straight beside a tall sturdy chair.

- Lightly grasp the chair with your fingertips.

- Raise one leg and foot off the ground to the side.

- Maintain your balance while standing on one leg.

- Hold for a count of ten seconds.

- Repeat with your other leg.

(continued)

Another simple balance activity is one that AARP president Jennie Chin Hansen recommends. You can do this at least twice a day: While brushing your teeth on the left side of your mouth, lift your left leg slightly and hold it up until you've finished. Then do the same with your right leg while brushing the right side.

For people who have never exercised

Even if you are a lifetime non-exerciser in good health, starting now can make you more resilient to illness, injury, or surgery in the future. Consider it an investment in your continued good health.

We can't tell you how active you should be to attain certain health benefits, but we can give you some research examples. Studies show that people who are active have a lower death rate than those who don't. And researchers have found that men in inactive occupations like bus and taxi drivers have a higher rate of heart disease than men in other occupations.

Except for starting with a warm-up, there is no recommended order to your activity routine. You can start with resistance training one day and balance exercises the next. And you don't have to do everything every day. You can even combine some activities like aerobic activity with resistance training (walking with hand or ankle weights, for example).

If you've never exercised before, talk to your doctor. Your doctor knows your medical conditions and surgical history—all of which should be taken into account before you begin any program. Based on your history, your doctor may recommend that you see an exercise professional or physical therapist to have an individualized, achievable program set up for you. Follow all of your doctor's recommendations—you'll get the most out of your activity program and be less prone to injury.

Keep in mind that some days will be better than others. Even if yesterday you were able to do ten minutes of aerobic activity, today you may only be able to do five minutes. It's normal for your tolerance to fluctuate. Do only what you can.

Getting Back to Being Active

Alexander is an eighty-year-old man with arthritis who always loved being active. In his younger days, he especially enjoyed pickle ball, a sport similar to badminton that uses paddles and perforated balls. Despite his arthritis he volunteered at local museums, traveled extensively, and especially enjoyed cruises. He eventually became less active, however, because of knee stiffness and pain. Alexander elected to have knee surgery.

After surgery, Alexander went to see a physical therapist, who designed an individualized program for his recovery. He dedicated himself to his rehabilitation and exercise program, and now he's back to his normal activity levels, and even playing pickle ball again.

Going for the Gold

Ray is a ninety-two-year-old who enjoyed competing in the Senior Olympics every year. A few months before he was scheduled to carry the Olympic torch in the opening ceremonies of the 2007 twenty-fifth anniversary of the Northern Virginia Olympics, he accidentally tripped while playing badminton, fracturing his right leg. He had to undergo upper leg surgery in June. At first he thought his torch-carrying dreams were over.

But Ray had set a goal for himself and intended to achieve it. He dedicated himself to his postsurgical physical and occupational therapy treatments. By keeping his primary goal in mind as well as setting smaller progress goals during his recovery, Ray was able to fulfill his dream of carrying the Olympic torch only three months after his surgery. He even went on to win gold medals in those games—in the softball throw and horseshoe events.

Skin Care: Looking Young on the Outside

Have you ever been guilty of looking at others your own age and thinking, *Surely I can't look that old*? Here's a story illustrating that very point:

A woman was sitting in the waiting room for her first appointment with a new dentist. She noticed his D.D.S. diploma, which bore his full name. Suddenly, she remembered a tall, handsome, dark-haired boy with the same name had been in her high school class some thirty-odd years ago. Could he be the same guy that she had had a secret crush on way back then? Upon seeing him, however, she quickly discarded any such thought. This balding, gray-haired man with the deeply lined face was way too old to have been her classmate.

After he examined her teeth, she asked him if he had attended West Park High School. He answered with pride, "Yes, I did. I'm a West Park Lion!" She asked him when he graduated. "Nineteen seventy! Why do you ask?" he answered. She exclaimed, "You were in my class!" He looked at her closely. Then he asked, "What did you teach?"

Feeling younger on the inside is wonderful. But if you are someone who wants to look younger on the outside, good skin care is essential. A good way to start is to avoid the sun.

Studies indicate that long-term exposure to the sun's ultraviolet (UV) rays can contribute to skin cancer, cataracts, and immune system suppression. Two types of UV rays reach the Earth's surface—UVA and UVB. UVB rays are stronger, but the weaker UVA rays are also known to be harmful. To avoid UV dangers as well as reduce the appearance of wrinkles and age spots, follow these tips.

1. Avoid sun exposure, especially between the hours of 10:00 a.m. and 4:00 p.m. when the sun's rays are strongest.
2. Use a moisturizing sunscreen with an SPF 30 or higher on your face, neck, hands, and any other body parts that are exposed to the sun. Apply fifteen to thirty minutes before going outside.
3. Reapply your sunscreen halfway through the day, as it will wear off.
4. Check your sunscreen's expiration date. Sunscreen without an expiration date has a shelf life of no more than three years, and exposure to extreme temperatures can further shorten its shelf life.
5. Wear a hat that has at least a three-inch brim all around (not just baseball cap styles).
6. If you live in a particularly sunny climate or have a personal or family history of skin cancer, have your doctor

or dermatologist closely inspect your skin at checkups. The key to successful skin cancer treatment is early detection. In between doctor's visits, have a family member help you check for any skin changes.

The cosmetics industry has been paying more attention to what older adults want. Many people over age sixty have expressed a desire for products that enhance, not combat, aging skin. Instead of looking like a model, older adults want to look like their best selves. Older role models in cosmetics commercials such as comedian Ellen DeGeneres and actor Diane Keaton reiterate this cultural shift.

Going a step further

As an alternative to plastic surgery, many older adults are using increasingly popular "medspas" (short for medical spas) that provide services available in a dermatologist's office but in a more luxurious, less clinical environment. Some examples of medspa services include microdermabrasion, injections of collagen fillers or wrinkle reducers such as Botox, removal of spider veins, and laser treatments that reduce age spots. Always check with your doctor before having any of these treatments, as they all have risks.

There are also treatments you can do at home. Several studies have shown that prescription-only Retin A cream improves the look of aging skin. Once again, it's prudent to check with your primary doctor before trying any at-home treatments. He/she may be able to recommend a dermatologist who can determine the best skin-care regimen for you.

Compensate When Necessary

If your daily functioning has been affected by an illness or injury, working with your doctor and a rehabilitation specialist can help ensure that you have all the tools you need to compensate for your lost motion or flexibility. Rehabilitation specialists can also help you manage flare-ups of conditions like arthritis. Along with prescribed exercises, they can recommend adaptive equipment or technologies that may help you remain as independent as possible.

Aside from standard equipment like canes, walkers, grab bars, and assistive devices and utensils (resources listed in Appendix A), there are many technologies that can be helpful. From something as simple as a daily automated phone call (in which a family member or emergency personnel is notified if you don't answer) to emerging technologies like "smart" medicine cabinets (which can monitor your medication schedule and even order refills) and "smart" homes (equipped with computers that help with your daily activities), your doctor and therapists can help you fill in the gaps. Many big companies are also developing sophisticated telehealth technologies, which deliver health-related services and information via telecommunications technologies. These technologies can provide a high level of at-home monitoring for people who cannot easily leave their homes or who have unstable medical conditions. People with diabetes, for example, can check their blood sugar with a special device that transmits the results directly to their doctor via telephone, allowing for instant medication adjustments. The same goes for people with heart disease or high blood pressure—telehealth technologies allow people to instantly send blood pressure results and even electrocardiograms (EKGs) to their doctors over phone lines.

One group in England has developed an especially sophisticated system for people with diabetes. A small home device administers more than a dozen tests normally performed in a doctor's office. Once the information is transmitted to the doctor, the patient is notified via cell phone of any abnormal results and the need for medical follow-up. This same group is partnering with a telecommunications company to develop a cell phone product for people with diabetes that scans grocery barcodes and indicates if a food product is safe and healthful.

We believe that when medical providers and patients are able to communicate crucial medical information in real time, better outcomes are likely. To this end, Erickson has been piloting telehealth technologies at select communities. A University of Missouri study demonstrated that technology adds to older adults' health monitoring. Over a period of two years, motion and bed sensor readings were tracked at an independent living retirement community. The goal was to correlate sensor readings to health events such as falls. Two of the case studies showed that sensor readings detected changes in the residents' conditions that were not detected by a traditional health assessment.

Electronic medical records (EMRs) are also a type of health technology, and Erickson has a fully-implemented EMR program throughout all communities nationwide. Residents can access their records securely via the Internet from anywhere in the world to check laboratory test results or even print a copy in the case of an urgent medical need while traveling.

Modify Your Home

You shouldn't change your habits to accommodate your home. If necessary, your home should be modified for your use. Depending on your functional limitations, you may need some or all of these suggestions.

Relocate your rooms. If your mobility is limited, move your bedroom and bathroom to the first floor to minimize stair climbing.

Install brighter lights. Even without severely impaired vision, installing brighter lights (by either buying more lamps or putting brighter bulbs in existing fixtures) can help you see better and avoid physical accidents. Just make sure you don't exceed the recommended wattage on your lamp, which is usually printed on a sticker near where you screw in the bulb.

Secure your rugs. Put anti-trip tape under area rugs and your bathmat if necessary. Place additional secured rugs on slippery surfaces like wood floors or linoleum.

Get a home safety monitoring device. Many home alarm systems are good for personal emergencies. You can also consider emergency notification devices that are worn around the wrist or neck, especially if you live alone.

Install grab bars. If you have trouble with balance or strength, grab bars are especially useful in the bathroom, where many falls occur.

Make necessary appliances and surfaces reachable. You may need a contractor to help you adjust the heights of your kitchen counters, cabinets, sinks, or other appliances.

Finally, consult with an occupational therapist; they are experts at home safety evaluation and modifications. If you believe you would benefit from this kind of consultation, you should discuss it with your doctor, who can make the appointment referral.

Create a Social Capital Group

At least nine million people in the U.S. need help with daily living activities like doing laundry, going to appointments, paying bills, or grocery shopping. Social capital groups can help.

Social capital groups are networks of people in your area with whom you "trade" talents or skills, based on everyone's needs. For example, if you can't drive but can sew or iron clothes, you could have a capable driver in the group take you where you need to go in exchange for ironing clothes or sewing. These types of groups are becoming more prevalent around the United States, and can be large or small, highly structured or more casual. Larger groups may need a full-time coordinator, but smaller groups can meet everyone's needs with the help of a few dedicated members.

To find such a group, start by talking to people in your neighborhood. Although older adults are most often in need of services, there are many time-pressed younger adults who may be willing to trade their talents and services, too. Places of worship are also good places to get linked with a social capital group.

Formal, highly organized social capital groups are a new trend, so you may have to search to find one, or start your own informal network in your area.

Secret #5: Know Your Weak Spots

The only way you truly know where to focus your efforts for keeping what you've got, getting back what you can, and compensating when necessary is to know your weak spots. You may already know some of them if you have, for example, high blood pressure or high cholesterol. But to truly assess all of your weak spots, you need a good medical home and thorough screening. Once you identify your weak spots, you can work on strengthening them. You may be able to prevent disasters like heart attacks, strokes, or falls. Although there are many health events that can sideline your functional abilities and independence, in this section we'll discuss some of the most common and preventable.

Heart Disease

According to the U.S. Department of Health and Human Services, heart disease is the leading cause of non-accidental death for people age fifty-five and up. Having heart disease can also lead to significant lifestyle changes and functional impairments. Studies show, however, that thousands of lives could be saved each year if people simply took some easy and inexpensive preventive health steps, like exercising and quitting smoking.

You may already know your risk of getting heart disease based on your family's history, but at the same time the more information you have, the better—like knowing your blood pressure and cholesterol levels. Very few people experience symptoms from having high blood pressure (hypertension or HBP) or high cholesterol. Get screened to keep track of your numbers.

You can't do much about some heart disease risk factors like family history and your age, but you have some control over many others. Both heart disease and stroke have many of the same risk factors, including hardening of the arteries (atherosclerosis), malfunctions of the heart's rhythm, and congestive heart failure.

Controllable Heart Disease and Stroke Risk Factors

Smoking

High blood pressure

High cholesterol

Diabetes

Being overweight or obese

Poor diet

An inactive lifestyle

Your blood pressure

Blood pressure is the force of blood pushing against your artery walls, measured in millimeters of mercury (mmHg). The first number (systolic pressure) measures the pressure when your heart beats. The second number (diastolic pressure) measures the pressure while your heart relaxes between beats.

High blood pressure is a serious condition that can lead to coronary heart disease, heart failure, stroke, kidney failure, and other health problems. About one in three adults in the United States has HBP, which usually has no symptoms. You can have it for years without knowing it. During this time, however, it can damage the heart, blood vessels, kidneys, and other parts of your body.

Knowing your blood pressure numbers is important, even when you're feeling fine. If your blood pressure is normal, you can work with your health care team to keep it that way. If your blood pressure is too high, you need treatment (which may involve lifestyle changes and/or medication) to prevent damage to your body's organs.

Blood pressure numbers at a glance:		
	Systolic	Diastolic
Normal blood pressure	less than 120	less than 80
High blood pressure	140 or more	90 or more
Pre-hypertension	120–139	80–89
High blood pressure is generally regarded as a reading of 140/90 mmHg or higher at two or more check-ups.		

Your cholesterol

Your cholesterol levels tend to rise as you get older. You are more likely to have high cholesterol if members of your family have it, if you are overweight, or if you eat a lot of fatty foods. There are usually no signs or symptoms that you have high blood cholesterol, but it can be measured with a blood test.

The types of cholesterol and other fats most commonly measured are high-density lipoproteins (HDLs or "good" cholesterol), low-density lipoproteins (LDLs or "bad" cholesterol), and triglycerides, a type of fat. Individual results vary, but it's better to have higher levels of HDLs and lower levels of LDLs and triglycerides.

Your total cholesterol reading is not as important as the balance among your individual component numbers. Only your doctor can determine if your numbers are ideal, based on your health and risk factors.

General Blood Cholesterol Guidelines

HDL cholesterol:
a reading greater than 60 milligrams per deciliter (mg/dl) can lend some protection against heart disease

LDL cholesterol:
less than 100 mg/dl is optimal

Triglycerides:
less than 150 mg/dl is optimal

How diabetes is related to heart disease

Having diabetes essentially means that your body cannot properly process sugar. You can have type 1, which results primarily from the body's failure to produce insulin (the hormone that allows glucose to enter and fuel the cells), or type 2, which results primarily from the body's failure to use insulin properly. Most Americans who are diagnosed with diabetes have type 2 diabetes.

At least 20 percent of adults over age sixty-five have diabetes, and at least 65 percent of people with diabetes die from heart disease or stroke. Over time, high blood sugar levels can lead to increased fatty deposits on the insides of blood vessel walls. These deposits may affect blood flow, increasing the chance of clogging and hardening of blood vessels (atherosclerosis). Atherosclerosis is one of the major causes of heart attacks and strokes in people with diabetes, so it's vitally important for people with diabetes to know their cholesterol profiles.

If you have type 1 or type 2 diabetes, watch your diet, know your cholesterol, and check your blood sugar levels as often as your doctor recommends. In addition, a glycosolated hemoglobin (A1c) blood test performed periodically can help your doctor determine how well your diabetes is controlled. If you don't have type 2 diabetes, research shows that making lifestyle changes like eating a better diet and exercising more can prevent or delay the onset of the disease.

Falls, Fractures, and Osteoporosis

According to the CDC, more than one-third of adults age sixty-five and older fall each year. Of those sixty-five-plus who fall, 20 to 30 percent suffer moderate to severe injuries—such as hip fractures or head traumas—that reduce mobility and independence and increase the risk of premature death. Hip fractures in particular can be devastating to older adults' health and functional abilities. CDC statistics also indicate that just 25 percent of hip-fracture patients over age fifty make a full recovery, 40 percent will require at least temporary nursing home care, and 24 percent die within twelve months.

Preventing falls helps to prevent fractures. Fall prevention strategies include:

- **Exercise regularly.** Along with aerobic exercise and resistance training, older adults should perform exercises that maintain or improve balance. Tai chi exercises are one example.

- **Have your medicines reviewed by your doctor.** Check both prescription and over-the-counter medicines. A thorough medicine review can help lessen side effects and interactions.

- **Have yearly eye exams.** Even slight changes in your vision can contribute to balance problems and falls.

- **Reduce fall hazards in your home.** Look for general clutter, loose cords, or rugs that are not secured to the floor. Have railings and banisters installed wherever appropriate.

Osteoporosis—a leading cause of fractures

Osteoporosis is a disease characterized by thinning, fragile bones that affects 55 percent of Americans age fifty and older. Approximately ten million people in the United States have osteoporosis, and another thirty-four million are estimated to have low bone mass (osteopenia), which places them at risk for developing osteoporosis. Eighty percent of those affected by osteoporosis are women. Men also contract the disease, but it usually develops later in life because men have larger bones and different hormonal factors affecting their bone density.

Despite these facts, osteoporosis often remains under-recognized and undertreated. You can't feel your bones thinning, so unless you undergo screenings, you won't know you have it. Often your first sign of osteoporosis is a fracture. One in two women and one in four men over age fifty will have an osteoporosis-related fracture in her/his remaining lifetime. Know your risk factors and get screened.

Many types of screening tests are available. The dual-energy x-ray absorptiometry (DXA or DEXA) scan is a low-dose x-ray exam that's considered the gold standard for

---

Risk Factors for Osteoporosis

Having a fracture after age fifty

Having low bone mass (osteopenia)

Being thin and/or having a small frame

A family history of osteoporosis or having a primary relative with a history of fracture

Estrogen deficiency as a result of menopause, especially early or surgically induced menopause

Vitamin D deficiency

Low calcium intake

Use of certain medications (examples: corticosteroids, chemotherapy, anticonvulsants, some diuretics)

Presence of certain chronic medical conditions (examples: Crohn's disease, Cushing's syndrome, celiac disease)

An inactive lifestyle

Smoking

Excessive alcohol use

diagnosing osteoporosis. DXA scans usually require a doctor's referral. You also have other screening options, like a portable quantitative ultrasound—a heel scan that assesses your bone strength. These machines along with portable DXA scanners are sometimes found in community pharmacies or at health fairs and don't usually require a doctor's referral.

After you are screened, follow up with your doctor to see if you need medication or other treatments for osteoporosis.

Assess Your Future Health

Studies have shown that a simple walking test may be a good predictor of your overall future health, disability, or even death. You should attempt the following assessment only if you are in good health and have your doctor's permission. Stop immediately if you experience chest pain, shortness of breath, dizziness, or significant fatigue.

The 400-meter (1/4-mile) walk test

This test should be performed on a level surface, such as a long corridor or a standard high school or college track. Walk for four hundred meters, or one time around a track, as fast as you can without running and time yourself. (Walking is defined as having at least one foot on the ground all the time.) Compare your results to the normal parameters in the chart below, adapted and summarized from a 2006 study by the National Institutes of Health:

Age	Men	Women
<66	Faster than 4 minutes 4 seconds	Faster than 4 minutes 40 seconds
66–74	Faster than 4 minutes 40 seconds	Faster than 5 minutes 25 seconds
75–84	Faster than 5 minutes 20 seconds	Faster than 6 minutes 10 seconds
85-plus	Faster than 6 minutes 10 seconds	Faster than 7 minutes 15 seconds

Get Started Now!

Government research shows that preventive health care practices could avert 100,000 deaths per year. Now that you have more information, you can make the right investments in your physical health—whether that's consciously choosing more heart-healthy foods rich in antioxidants or making the commitment to walk regularly with your spouse or a friend. If you haven't already, make it a priority to "find your team," beginning with a personal physician who makes your health care a priority, and stay up-to-date with all of your screenings. It's never too late to start.

CHAPTER THREE
Age Is a State of Mind

"Ninety percent of the game is half mental."

—Yogi Berra

Legendary baseball players have much wisdom to share about the aging process and your brain. Satchel Paige, one of the oldest performers in major league baseball (some sources estimate that he played well into his fifties) once said, "Age is mind over matter. If you don't mind, it doesn't matter."

To paraphrase, training your mind is critical for successful aging because your mind is where you develop the resilience that helps with the inevitable challenges of life. Despite physical aging processes, including changes in your brain, you can take steps to keep your mind sharp.

How Your Brain Ages

Until the 1980s, the scientific community believed that brain aging was associated primarily with the loss of brain cells (neurons). It was generally believed that people lost thousands or even millions of neurons daily beginning at birth. Better technology, however, has led to the discovery that healthy aging brains may have essentially the same number of neurons as younger brains, although some *larger* neurons may decrease. These neurons can only multiply forty to sixty times before tiring out forever, and they tend to regenerate at a slower rate than other cells.

Research shows that brain aging is largely about topographical changes. That three-pound organ in your head may gradually lose from 5 percent to 10 percent of its weight by the time you reach age ninety (possibly due to the loss of large neurons). The grooves on your brain's surface may widen, and chemical reactions may change due to physical changes in neuron connections.

So what exactly causes the changes in your brain function, like memory loss, as you age? The most recent research points to changes in the efficiency of your brain's chemical connections. In addition, amounts of certain brain chemicals may also decrease, affecting your processing speed.

Research has also shown that some mental activity decline may be attributed to a general slowing down of your lifestyle, or falling into comfortable, "old dog" routines that form during your middle and older years.

Although many other brain changes can occur with different disease processes, like strokes or dementia, our focus in this chapter will be on the healthy aging brain.

Your Mind's Abilities: What Does and Doesn't Change

As you age, it may seem that your memory is failing when you keep forgetting your keys or what you had for dinner last week. But there are other functions besides memory going on in your brain that may be changing—like your reasoning and processing speed.

Reasoning

Your reasoning and the ability to make logical connections slow down as you age. It might take you longer, for example, to figure out a bus schedule—at what intervals the buses run, when rush hour is defined on the schedule, and so on. Decreased reasoning ability may also affect the rationality of your decision making—causing you to feel frustrated or fearful about making major decisions. Or you may find that it takes you a longer time to reach important decisions because you can't sort out the details. You can, however, train your reasoning to be more sound with the exercises later in this chapter.

Processing speed

Processing speed relates to how fast you can translate information into action. When your processing speed slows down, your reaction times (to jokes, clever word twists, and even changing traffic lights) slow down, too. You can also train your processing speed to be more efficient with the exercises later in this chapter.

Memory

There are many different kinds of memory, and they all work in slightly different fashions. All memory is created by the connections among your brain's neurons. How the neurons connect determines where the memory is stored and how the information is retrieved.

Short-term and long-term memory

Much research has been conducted on short- and long-term memory, and there is considerable debate about which is which and how each works. Your short-term memory is also called your "working" memory: what you retain for short periods of time (twenty to thirty seconds) while using or processing information. Whenever you see, hear, or receive information, your neurons connect in a certain pattern. When you remember that same information, the neurons reconnect in that same pattern. Short-term memories are stored in an area of your brain called the hippocampus. In Alzheimer's disease, the hippocampus is one of the first areas affected; that's why Alzheimer's sufferers lose their short-term memories first (they may remember their spouse but not their newborn grandchild).

Long-term memory can be considered as either your behavioral or cognitive functions. Behavioral functions are those like how to ride a bike or how to cook a favorite dish. Very often these types of memories stay intact as you age, even in the presence of dementia. Cognitive functions are your thinking abilities—understanding ideas, information, and processes. Where your brain stores long-term memories is largely unknown, although many scientists believe they are stored in an area called the anterior cingulate cortex. Your brain is like a filing system—some information is not readily retrievable (like information you throw in the trash or store in a "miscellaneous" desk file) and some is easily accessible (like information filed in easily accessed, well-labeled file folders). Some cognitive memories may be harder to access as you age depending on where they're stored. And your neurons may reconnect differently when you access your long-term memory; that may be why some details may be incomplete or the memory of a particular event seems "fuzzy."

Recall and recognition memory

Both short- and long-term memory are general categories. Recall and recognition memory are specific types that can be part of either short- or long-term memory depending upon where the particular information is stored.

Many older adults are concerned about these two specific types of memory. Your recall memory is the set of processes that help you retrieve certain information (like the name of your friend's neighbor who you met last week). Struggling to name something that is right on the tip of your tongue is also your recall memory at work.

Your recognition memory is the set of complex processes that allows you to pick out your friend's neighbor's name from a list, even if you couldn't produce the name otherwise. The good news is that your recognition memory stays mostly intact as you age. Your recall memory, however, may not be as keen.

An Illustration of How Your Mind Changes

Burt is in his eighties. He knows that he remembers some things well and forgets others. For example, although he's talked with her before, he can't recall his interviewer's name.

When asked about his working years, however, Burt can give precise details. "I retired in 1984. I used to work in the government building at 17th and Constitution Avenue. That was the main Navy building—it's not there anymore. While working there, I used to run regularly at the nearby YMCA track. That track had a slant to it, and I swear the leg that used to hit the higher portion of the track is now shorter than my other leg. My doctor also noticed the difference!"

Burt has demonstrated several of his mind's abilities: the ability to process and tell a story; the ability to make an educated guess about having one leg shorter than the other; and the ability to remember and relate information from his long-term memory.

Burt has also demonstrated the difference between recall and recognition memory—although he may have trouble recalling the name of his interviewer, he knows that he recognizes her.

Test Your Recognition and Recall Memory

The Hopkins Verbal Learning Test helps assess your recognition and recall memory. This is an adapted version of the test.

Directions for taking the test:

Step 1: Enlist the assistance of a friend or family member.

Step 2: Give your assistant the list in *Part A – Free Recall* to read to you—at two-second intervals per word.

Step 3: Repeat as many of the words back as possible. Your assistant should be checking off the words under each trial as you say them.

Step 4: Repeat steps 2-3 with two more attempts (trials) at repeating all the words back.

Step 5: Have your assistant read to you the words in *Part B – Recognition.* You indicate whether or not each word was in the original list from Part A.

Step 6: *Part C – Delayed Recall:* (not a part of your score). If you'd like, you can try to repeat the words back to your assistant now, without help.

Part A: Free Memory Recall Part C: Delayed Recall Memory

	Trial 1	Trial 2	Trial 3	Delayed trial
lion	❏	❏	❏	❏
skirt	❏	❏	❏	❏
pistol	❏	❏	❏	❏
horse	❏	❏	❏	❏
blouse	❏	❏	❏	❏
bomb	❏	❏	❏	❏
flute	❏	❏	❏	❏
tiger	❏	❏	❏	❏

violin	❑	❑	❑	❑
shoes	❑	❑	❑	❑
rifle	❑	❑	❑	❑
clarinet	❑	❑	❑	❑

Part B – Recognition Memory

Mark an X for Yes or No beside each word to indicate response.

Was this word part of the original list I read to you?

apple	❑ Yes	❑ No
deer	❑ Yes	❑ No
lion	❑ Yes	❑ No
skirt	❑ Yes	❑ No
pistol	❑ Yes	❑ No
bullet	❑ Yes	❑ No
furnace	❑ Yes	❑ No
horse	❑ Yes	❑ No
blouse	❑ Yes	❑ No
bomb	❑ Yes	❑ No
flute	❑ Yes	❑ No
guitar	❑ Yes	❑ No
roof	❑ Yes	❑ No
tiger	❑ Yes	❑ No
ocean	❑ Yes	❑ No
cello	❑ Yes	❑ No
violin	❑ Yes	❑ No
music	❑ Yes	❑ No
harp	❑ Yes	❑ No
shoes	❑ Yes	❑ No
rifle	❑ Yes	❑ No
tree	❑ Yes	❑ No
clarinet	❑ Yes	❑ No

Step 7: Scoring.

Ask your assistant to add up the number you got right in each of the three parts. A perfect score in the first part would be 36. A perfect score in the second part would be 24. A perfect score in the third part would be 12.

If you are younger than fifty-five years of age . . .

Part I:

A score of 33 – 36: Your free memory recall is great!

A score of 25 – 32: This is where most of your peers seem to be, so you're fine.

A score of 15 – 24: Consider exercising your mind more.

A score of less than 15: Consult your doctor for further discussion.

Part II:

A score of 24: Your recognition memory is terrific!

A score of 20-23: Your recognition memory seems fine.

A score of less than 20: Consider some exercises.

Part III:

A score of 12: Your delayed recall memory is terrific!

A score of 10-11: Your recognition memory seems fine.

A score of less than 10: Consider some exercises.

If you are between fifty-five to sixty-nine years of age . . .

Part I:

A score of 32-36: Your free recall memory recall is great!

A score of 23-31: This is where most of your peers seem to be, so you're fine.

A score of 15-22: Consider exercising your mind more.

A score of less than 15: Consult your doctor for further discussion.

Part II:
A score of 24: Your recognition memory is terrific!
A score of 20-23: Your recognition memory seems fine.
A score of less than 20: Consider some exercises.

Part III:
A score of 12: Your delayed recall memory is terrific!
A score of 8-11: Your recognition memory seems fine.
A score of less than 10: Consider some exercises.

If you are over seventy years of age . . .

Part I:
A score of 32-36: Your free recall memory is great!
A score of 19-31: This is where most of your peers seem to be, so you're fine.
A score of 15-18: Consider exercising your mind more.
A score of less than 15: Consult your doctor for further discussion.

Part II:
A score of 24: Your recognition memory is terrific!
A score of 20-23: Your recognition memory seems fine.
A score of less than 20: Consider some brain exercises.

Part III:
A score of 11-12: Your delayed recall memory is terrific!
A score of 6-10: Your recognition memory seems fine.
A score of less than 6: Consider some brain exercises.

Keep What You've Got

Even if you're happy with how your mind currently operates, research shows that it takes practice exercising your brain to keep your neuron connections flexible and your memory, processing speed, and reasoning abilities sharp. And there may be added benefits: Research shows that leisure activities involving physical, mental, and social stimulation all offer some protection against developing dementia, but activities that combine all three types of stimulation offer the greatest benefits.

Secret #6: Stay Curious

Although doing crossword puzzles and numbers games like Sudoku may seem like a vigorous workout for your brain, there is little research supporting mental benefits of playing these games on a daily basis. Instead, evidence shows that doing the same activities every day may make your mind stagnant. It's better to stay curious and participate in a variety of activities and experiences.

A study published in the *New England Journal of Medicine* found that people who participated in interactive activities like board games, square dancing, and playing musical instruments tended to maintain their mental abilities. The study also found that fewer people who engaged in these types of activities developed dementia than those who didn't.

The Concept of Brain Plasticity

Staying curious and participating in a variety of interactive pursuits helps you maintain your brain's "plasticity," your brain's ability to rearrange the connections between its neurons. It is the foundation of memory formation and learning processes, and it can help compensate for brain damage by allowing the brain to create new networks of neurons.

How to Know If You're Stuck in a Routine

Most people have some kind of daily routine. You need some routines to stay organized and provide structure in your life. Too much routine, however, can cause your mind to stagnate.

Write down what you do every day (use an hourly schedule, so you don't skip anything). After two weeks, review your schedule. Do you see a pattern with little variation? If so, start by varying one or two aspects of your routine every week; then increase your variation frequency until you are trying something new every day. Varying your routine and trying new things help your brain forge new pathways and keep you sharp.

His Routines Disrupted an Entire Town

Eighteenth-century philosopher Immanuel Kant lived in a time when clocks were set manually. Legend has it that every day at the same time he would walk past the same shops to the same cafe for breakfast. He ran the same daily errands at the same times each day. He worked at home and taught students on a rigid schedule. Kant supposedly had such a reliable routine that his fellow townspeople used to set their clocks according to his rigorous schedule.

One day, however, Kant became engrossed in a book. He ended up spending two weeks at home reading it. The result? It is said that the entire town was thrown into disarray because they were so accustomed to relying on him to determine the time.

How Can You Spice Up Your Daily Life?

As we said earlier, research shows that interactive activities benefit your brain the most. These types of activities help your brain exercise several pathways at once and keep your connections working efficiently. Most activities involve interacting with others, exchanging new ideas, or learning a new skill. Some examples:

Dance

Popular ones for older adults are square dancing and ballroom dancing, both of which require partners. You are training your brain to learn new movements while interacting verbally.

Actively participate in book discussion groups, or discuss new books or magazine articles with friends.

This easy and inexpensive activity sharpens your mind because it helps you formulate and communicate new ideas.

Learn a new language.

Research shows that hearing new accents, practicing different grammatical structures, and uttering new sounds triggers your brain to stay sharp. Try one of the world's easiest languages called Bahasa, spoken in Indonesia and Malaysia. Or, plan a trip to a foreign country and challenge yourself to learn the language.

Learn a musical instrument.

Learning to play (or practicing one you've already learned) keeps your mind in shape by hearing new sounds, seeing and interpreting musical notes, and synchronizing hand-eye coordination.

Volunteer your brain for your community.

Find a way to share your knowledge and experience for the benefit of others. A Johns Hopkins School of Medicine study showed that older adults who participated in Experience Corps, a nationwide program in which adults age fifty-five and over tutor and mentor schoolchildren, had increased cognitive abilities. Brain scans documented the increased mental activity in study participants.

Experience new ways to vacation.

Instead of your usual summer trip, seek out new experiences with an educational travel organization like Elderhostel or a senior-friendly travel group like Grand Circle Travel.

Examples of other activities that have been associated with sharper minds are acting, painting/art, quilting, photography, and even surfing the Internet. Most of the above activities have been scientifically studied with regard to their brain benefits. Keep in mind, however, that any activity can be beneficial as long as it's something new to you.

A Simple Way to Stay Curious

Ellen is a sixty-eight-year-old former educator. She enjoys her daily crossword puzzle and other games, and she likes her weekly routines. She knows, however, that to keep out of a rut she needs to try something new once in a while.

Ellen keeps it simple. Although she tends to go to many of the same places each week, she seeks out new ways to get to her destinations. She looks at maps and traces out new routes. In this way Ellen enjoys new scenery, and it keeps her extra alert behind the wheel. And getting lost occasionally is not a bad thing; by using her maps and sometimes asking people for directions, Ellen is training herself to be a champion problem solver.

Varying your activities doesn't have to be a complex venture. Take Ellen's example, or try something like shopping at a different store once a month.

One Skill Enhances Another

Louise is eighty-two years old. She used to work as a United Nations translator and is fluent in French, German, and Italian. She practices her language skills regularly, and along with making her an excellent communicator, Louise found that this brain exercise has yielded added benefits in her daily life.

Louise elaborates: "Practicing languages, both reading and speaking, is what keeps me sharp. It helps me keep other things straight in my head. Every week, when I go to the grocery store, I'm able to keep a running dollar tally of the items in my cart without a calculator. By the time I reach check-out, I know to the dollar, and sometimes even to the penny, what I'll be paying."

Beware of One-way Learning

Some activities might seem like a good idea for sharpening your mind, but research shows otherwise. An example is taking college classes or attending lectures. Simply listening to a lecture, whether in a formal class or otherwise, does not provide enough brain stimulation to positively impact mental fitness.

If you want to take classes or attend lectures, look for those that are discussion-based and interactive. If you take a class that doesn't offer discussion or activities, set aside time to talk about the subject matter with friends or family.

Get Back What You Can

If you want your brain to function as well as it did in your younger days, you've got to work at it. Fortunately, research is increasingly providing proof about ways to achieve your goals, no matter what your age or health status.

The Erickson Foundation compared a case-matched sample of Erickson residents to a representative sample of older adults enrolled in the nationwide Health and Retirement Study (HRS). Despite having more chronic conditions than their HRS counterparts, Erickson residents reported being in better health and experiencing less depression. In general, they felt happier. We believe that these results are due, in part, to Erickson residents' active participation in campus activities and social interaction.

Secret #7: Sharpen Your Mind

No matter how old you are or how forgetful you've become, there are ways you can regain some of your mental sharpness. More and more research studies are showing that you can reprogram your brain to function better. One way to do this is by using brain exercises.

Formal brain exercises, like those developed by Nintendo, Advanced Brain Technologies, PositScience, Quixit, CogniFit, and many others, can be effective for some users. One program developed by PositScience has been shown in several research studies to shave ten years off of a seventy-five-year-old's brain age. Although several of these products look and sound like simple video games, they can be expensive. Individual users have to pay about $395 for the PositScience program, for example.

To help our residents get more physically active at Erickson communities, we tried the Nintendo Wii system, with an excellent response. We therefore decided to give Nintendo's Brain Age a try. Although not yet proven scientifically to better your brain function, and the "brain ages" that the game assigns to you need to be taken with a grain of salt, Brain

Age is nevertheless a big hit in Japan, where many people carry the portable game and play throughout the day, hoping to improve their brain age. Many of our residents enjoy the system, and one eighty-two-year old resident had this to say: "When I first started playing, the system scored my brain age as eighty. I played it every day for a week and now my brain age is sixty-seven. I think the game helps me concentrate better."

Another 2008 study from researchers at the University of Illinois showed that playing complex video games may improve older adults' thinking abilities and help them juggle multiple tasks.

There are other, informal brain exercises that can provide you with the same kind of targeted brain training for a lot less money. Targeted brain training means that the exercises are designed for a specific purpose (like improving memory) in the same way that targeted physical exercises concentrate on certain muscle groups.

Brain Exercises to Practice at Home

Some of the following exercises were developed by Dr. George Rebok, a Johns Hopkins professor and world-renowned expert on older adults' mental health, and his colleagues.

Improve your memory skills

These tips are useful for improving all types of memory.

Step one: Pay attention. It's common sense, but you tend to remember what you pay attention to. Example: When you meet someone new, you may be so focused on what to say that you don't pay attention to his/her name. Repeat the person's name to yourself a few times or out loud ("It's nice to meet you, Bob"), and you'll be less likely to forget it next time.

The following steps can be remembered by the acronym, "M.O.V.A."

Step two: M = Meaningfulness. Make what you want to remember meaningful. Example: If you read something important or interesting, discuss it with someone, or better yet, several people. Talking about it will help the information stick in your memory.

Step three: O = Organization. Group information into natural categories. Example: When planning a trip to the grocery store, group needed items into categories that make the most sense to you—either by product type (e.g., produce, dairy, meats), meals planned for the week, or the store's layout. Then try to shop without consulting your list. Organization works well with any large amount of information you need to remember—instructions for setting up your computer, for example.

Step four: V = Visualization. See the information in your mind. Visualization lends meaning to the object or information to be remembered and allows the creation of a mental picture that helps with later recall. Example: A good way to practice visualization is to draw or write down what you see. Sharpen your skills by drawing a penny from memory, or anything else you've seen thousands of times, like a building you pass by every day.

Step five: A = Association. Associate new information with what you already know. Example: If you want to remember a painting to describe to someone, start by concentrating on the painting's elements individually. Associate each element with something familiar—if there's a person wearing a hat, think about a favorite hat you've owned. Or if there's a tree, associate it with the tree outside your window. Then try describing the painting in detail.

A Meaningful First Love

Dr. Terry Bard, a professor and clinical psychologist from Harvard Medical School, says that most people, no matter how young or old, recall the name of their first girlfriend or boyfriend. Why? Because for most, the experience of your first girlfriend or boyfriend is associated with many meaningful memories and may have formed a model for future relationships in your life.

Dr. Bard remembers his first girlfriend, Linda, from when he was thirteen. When he was in his early twenties, he looked her up and called. She asked, "Who IS this?" and Dr. Bard answered, "Your first love." After a ten-second pause she said, "Terry . . . ?" Linda remembered Terry because of their shared and meaningful experience.

Strong Associations Spark Memory

Dr. Bard relates another story illustrating how strong associations can jog your memory.

"I attended my twenty-fifth high school reunion recently. Someone asked me beforehand if I knew a 'Richard Moose' who graduated in my class, I said, 'no'.

"As I walked down the hallway at the reunion, however, I saw a man coming toward me. I was suddenly flooded with remembered experiences and associations—his large and chunky frame, his daredevil attitude, his unusual way of crashing into the classroom—all of which came to me in seconds. Then, without any conscious thought I heard myself calling out his nickname, 'MOOOOOSE!' I guess I remembered him, after all."

Sharpen your reasoning skills

Sharpening your reasoning skills helps you solve problems. Look for patterns and logic when figuring something out. Example: Look at a bus or train schedule, and calculate the time between departures. Write up a medication schedule for yourself or someone else.

- Other activities that can help you think "on your feet" and solve problems:

- Volunteer at a museum, airport, or library customer service or "help" desk.

- Sign up to be a clinical actor at a local teaching hospital. As a clinical actor you play the part of a patient to help teach medical students and interns (they especially like older adults in these roles).

- Work part-time at a local business's reception desk.

Increase your processing speed

Processing speed (how quickly you mentally digest information) has been shown to slow down as you age, largely because your processing speed is dependent upon the efficiency of your brain connections. In addition, if your processing speed slows down, so do your memory and reasoning.

Processing speed has always been an issue for older drivers, in particular. Researchers have found that it takes more than good vision to avoid accidents. A test called the "useful field of view" was developed to assess visual processing speed. Useful field of view is the area from which you can extract information in a single glance without moving your head or eyes. Studies show that people who have a reduced useful field of view are more likely to fall and are six times more likely to be involved in an auto accident. Training programs designed to improve your visual processing speed are available for purchase through PositScience.

Improving your brain doesn't have to be formal or expensive. Simply walking with a friend while discussing a book not only gives you some physical exercise, it exercises your memory, reasoning, and processing speed as well.

When it comes to brain exercises, always practice, practice, practice. The payoff is worth it. Just a few weeks of brain training has been shown to have beneficial effects for months and possibly years.

Sharpen Your Senses to Sharpen Your Mind

When you are young, you learn largely through your sensory experiences—sight, sound, smell, taste, and touch. As you incorporate new knowledge, your brain's neurons get wired and rewired repeatedly, increasing your brain's plasticity.

Comparisons of brain scans show a high amount of plasticity until puberty, then a decline in the post-puberty years. In even later years, especially if you get mired in the same routines, the brain becomes hard-wired, or less elastic. Hence the wisdom behind the old saying, "You can't teach an old dog new tricks."

All of your senses decline somewhat with age. Your vision and hearing are less acute, your ability to taste and smell subtle flavors and aromas declines, and you even lose some sense of touch—especially your awareness of temperature and vibration.

The brain is stimulated each time you see, hear, or activate any of your senses. It's the same as your body being stimulated each time you exercise a major muscle group; so a decline in your senses means a decline in your brain's daily workout. If your brain is not getting a good workout from your five senses, overall mental fitness decreases.

To know where to focus your sensory-improvement efforts, get tested. Your senses may be changing at such a gradual rate that you may not notice deficits. Hearing and vision changes are the most dramatic, but all senses can be affected by aging. Fortunately, you can compensate for many of these changes by using equipment such as glasses and hearing aids or by making minor lifestyle changes.

Your vision

Your eye structure changes with aging. The cornea, the transparent surface of your eye, becomes less sensitive, so injuries may not be noticed. By the time you turn sixty, your pupils decrease to about one-third of the size they were when you were twenty, and they may react more slowly in response to darkness or bright light. The lens becomes yellowed, less flexible, and slightly cloudy. The fat pads supporting the eye decrease, and the eye sinks back into the socket. The eye muscles become less able to fully rotate the eye.

All of these changes mean that the sharpness of your vision may gradually decline. Glasses or contact lenses can help correct age-related vision changes. Almost everyone older than age fifty-five needs glasses at least part of the time, however, the amount of change is not universal. Only 15 percent to 20 percent of older people have bad enough vision to impair driving ability, and only 5 percent become unable to read. The most common problem is difficulty focusing the eyes (a condition called presbyopia).

Have your glasses or contacts checked to ensure that they are adequate for your changing vision. Having your eyes examined regularly can also detect the gradual onset of conditions like cataracts and glaucoma.

Your hearing

Your hearing may start to decline as early as your forties or fifties, possibly due to changes in the auditory nerve. In addition, the brain may have a slightly decreased ability to process or translate sounds into meaningful information. Impacted ear wax is another cause of hearing difficulties and is more common with increasing age.

It is estimated that 30 percent of all people over age sixty-five have significant hearing impairment. You may find it more difficult to hear sounds in higher registers, and you may strain to follow the words of people who speak rapidly. Hearing tests can determine what kind of hearing loss you have and which assistive devices may help.

Your senses of smell and taste

The senses of taste and smell interact closely. Most of your taste sense is dependent on your sense of smell. The sense of smell begins at nerve receptors high in the membranes of the nose and may diminish, especially after age seventy. This decline may be related to the loss of nerve endings in the nose.

Studies about age-related causes of decreased sense of taste and smell have conflicting results. Some studies have indicated that normal aging by itself produces very little change in taste and smell. Rather, changes may be related to diseases, smoking, the presence of artificial dental work, and/or environmental exposures over a lifetime.

Believe it or not, there are ways to test your senses of smell and taste. Scientists have developed an easily administered "scratch-and-sniff" test to evaluate the sense of smell, and there are substances that can be applied to different areas of your tongue to test taste.

Unfortunately, unless your losses of smell and taste are related to a particular modifiable condition, like the presence of polyps, ill-fitting dental work, or to certain medications, there's not much you can do to restore these senses.

Sometimes changes in the way food is prepared, such as a change in spices, may help.

Your sense of touch

The skin, muscles, tendons, joints, and internal organs have receptors that detect touch, temperature, or pain. Many studies have shown that with aging, you may have reduced or changed sensations, especially of pain, vibration, cold, heat, pressure, and touch. It is often hard to determine if these changes are related to aging itself or to the disorders that occur more often in older adults. It may be that some of the normal changes of aging are caused by decreased blood flow to the touch receptors or to the brain and spinal cord. Minor dietary deficiencies, such as decreased thiamine levels, may also be a cause.

Medications, brain surgery, brain disorders, and nerve damage from trauma or chronic diseases such as diabetes can change your interpretation of a sensation without changing your awareness of it. For example, you may feel and recognize a painful sensation, but it may not bother you.

Regardless of the cause, many people experience changes in touch-related sensations as they age. To increase safety, make allowances for these changes.

- Limit the maximum water temperature in your house (there is an adjustment on the water heater) to reduce the risk of burns.

- Look at your thermometer to decide how to dress rather than waiting until you feel overheated or chilled.

- Inspect your skin (especially your feet) for injuries, and if you find an injury, treat it. Don't assume that just because an area is not painful, the injury is not significant.

The Brain/Body Connection

Keeping your body fit through diet and activity benefits your mental fitness. Along with keeping health conditions that directly affect your brain at bay (like diabetes and strokes), research demonstrates improvement in older adults' mental functioning with a good diet and exercise.

Feeding yourself a nutritious diet as discussed in Chapter Two can stave off mental decline, and some studies show that adhering to a Mediterranean diet (especially one rich in fish) may reduce your risk of Alzheimer's disease by up to 60 percent.

One study found particular brain benefits for sixty- to eighty-year-olds who walked three times a week for six months. Compared to their non-exercising counterparts, the walkers had more cognitive flexibility and even increased brain volumes equivalent to adults who were up to three years younger. Even more compelling—studies have revealed that older adults may get greater overall benefits from exercise than younger adults.

Along with better overall brain function, exercise has been proven to be the biological equivalent of antidepressants when it comes to improving your mood. Increased activity stimulates your brain's mood center (the hippocampus, also the hub of short-term memory) and facilitates the release of chemicals like dopamine, serotonin, and norepinephrine—all essential for stable mood functions. Reducing your risk of depression not only helps you function better in your daily life, it may also benefit you in the long run: Research indicates that recurring bouts of depression may be associated with an increased risk of dementia.

Because of sophisticated technology and a better understanding of how our brains work, scientists are closer to understanding why exercise can have such profound positive results for older adults. Whenever a muscle is exercised, it sends out chemical messages that travel to the brain, facilitating the release of brain-derived neurotrophic factor, or BDNF. Research about BDNF suggests that it may be responsible for stimulating neuron growth as well as facilitating efficient connections among existing neurons.

On a broader level, exercise helps improve your blood flow by keeping your vascular system in better shape. A well-functioning vascular system can help you avoid heart disease, strokes, and complications of diabetes. Research shows that strokes and diabetes are associated with a higher risk of dementia.

Even a small amount of physical activity has been shown to have benefits for people who already have cognitive problems. One study revealed that participants who exercised (mainly in the form of brisk walking) only a couple of hours each week for six months showed improvements in their mental processing. More important, these improvements persisted for twelve months even after the activity stopped.

Teaching an Old Dog New Tricks

A group of researchers wanted to find out if it was actually possible to teach an old dog new tricks. They tested aging beagles by having them attempt to solve complex problems finding dog treats. One group of beagles received no special treatment; the other group received diets fortified with fruits and vegetables, more daily exercise, and plenty of time to play with other dogs and interesting toys. The beagles who received special treatment had a much easier time learning their new tricks.

Of Mice and Memory

Throughout their lives, mice and other rodents develop new cells in the area of their brains responsible for learning and memory. In one study, a group of mice was raised in a standard cage environment and another group was raised in an enriched environment. The enriched environment was larger, contained more mice, had tunnels, toys, and exercise equipment. Mice living in this environment also received "treats" of cheese, crackers, and fruit in addition to their regular mouse chow. Study results showed that the enriched mice developed more learning and memory brain cells than the mice raised in standard environments. A companion study showed that aging mice that were moved to the enriched environment also developed more brain cells than aging mice in standard environments.

Science at Work: Exercise and Coping with Grief

For over fifty-six years, Ken was married to Bonnie, the love of his life. They had raised a family and were enjoying each other's company in retirement with many friends and activities.

After a fall at home, however, Bonnie's health deteriorated. She developed complications, including dementia and pneumonia, and eventually died. Because Ken had spent countless hours caring for Bonnie, his health had also deteriorated. He attended some grief counseling sessions and learned that he was exhibiting signs of depression, like a poor appetite, difficulty sleeping, and a lack of desire to go out of his apartment or interact with anyone.

Ken knew he had to do something to get some relief from his crushing grief.

Ken started walking. At first, walking felt like a chore. Even walking a mile seemed to take five hours and left him exhausted. But gradually he noticed an improvement in his appetite and he was sleeping better, so he kept walking—sometimes up to three times a day. He began to talk more to people he saw along his route. Talking about his loss helped him feel less burdened, and he decided to write a tribute to his late wife, although he felt incapable at first of completing such an ambitious task. He eventually enlisted the aid of family and friends and was able to complete a written memorial, which he had bound and printed.

Ken's decision to champion his own health simply by walking served to improve his physical health and helped him strengthen his mind and spirit.

Compensate When Necessary

Even in the absence of a stroke or other illness, some people have persistent memory problems. You can, however, learn some new habits and tricks to help you adapt to your memory gaps.

Write Everything Down

Get comfortable keeping lists of what you need to remember every day, but be consistent in your methods. If you write a list, keep it in the same place. If you use a personal data assistant or other electronic device, be sure it's always within reach. If you use calendars, transfer all information to one master calendar.

Create Workaround Systems

Despite meticulous list-writing, there may be certain things you frequently forget. Do you often lock yourself out of your house or car? Hide a set of keys or give copies to a nearby friend or family member. Do you frequently misplace your wallet, cell phone, or keys? Tracking products are available ranging from simple keychain finders to more complex receiver systems that allow you to "tag" a number of items to locate with the press of a button. Always forgetting appointments? Set alarms on your cell phone or computer, or keep a small appointment book with you and update it daily. Do you forget important information or tasks that come up throughout your day? Keep paper or a small notebook with you at all times. Write down what you need to remember and then deal with the information at the end of your day— either transfer it to your master calendar or telephone book, update your cell phone alarms, or do other tasks like make necessary phone calls.

Don't Expect Perfection

After retiring from a lifelong accounting career, Mike worked part-time at a local business helping people prepare their tax returns. In his spare time, he stayed active by swimming and skiing, despite being over seventy years old. With his wife of over fifty years, Suzanne, Mike was enjoying life to the fullest.

Then Mike suddenly had a stroke. For several months he lost most of his memory, even forgetting the names of his wife and children. Mike required months of extensive rehabilitation, including physical, occupational, and speech therapy. Now, over five years later, Mike can communicate better, but he will always have problems remembering certain things. He has learned to appreciate those things he was able to recover and to be patient with himself, knowing that he can't necessarily do everything he used to do before his stroke.

Keep Your Sense of Humor

Albert is a seventy-two-year-old who used to own a small motel chain. Operating his businesses required a keen attention to detail, and Albert learned how to manage many tasks at once—mainly by writing everything down in lists.

After he retired, Albert developed several medical conditions. The complexity of his health status means that he sees several doctors and sometimes has multiple appointments each week. He keeps his schedule organized by noting all appointments on a small monthly calendar, and he's never missed a single appointment.

But nobody's perfect, and although Albert has one important aspect of his life well organized, he sometimes forgets other, equally important things. Several months ago, Albert received some Social Security documents in the mail. He sequestered them in a safe hiding place but neglected to tell anyone or notate where they were. He still can't find the documents. But Albert laughs about his situation, "It seems I've lost those papers and part of my mind with them!"

Our Main Message on Mental Fitness

Your mental fitness is not all about the state of your memory. It includes your reasoning and processing speed as well as maintenance of your five senses. Your mind and body are one, and making good lifestyle choices is the best thing you can do for your memory and your mood. The most important things you can do for your brain are to stimulate it with a good diet and exercise, learn new activities, engage in social activities, vary your routines, and most important—have fun.

CHAPTER FOUR

Socially Engaged

"Interdependence is and ought to be as much the ideal of man as self-sufficiency. Man is a social being."

—Mahatma Gandhi

Your social health is closely related to your mental fitness. After all, if you are socially active, you are probably already engaging in the types of interactive activities that keep your brain working efficiently. Being socially active does not necessarily mean having your calendar chock full of dates with different friends every night of the week. Going to church or having dinner with your family both count as good social activities because you are interacting in both situations. A government survey, however, showed that Americans age sixty-five and older spend up to half of their leisure time watching television.

Keep What You've Got

We told you in Chapter One about the University of Chicago study in which three out of four adults ages fifty-seven to eighty-five participated in at least one social activity per week, and many had more good friends and family relationships than younger adults. Some people stay quite busy trying new things and meeting new people, and research indicates that maintaining these contacts with family or close friends is one of the best ways to combat loneliness and isolation. If you currently see your family and friends regularly, you're on the right track. At the same time, however, you should take steps to avoid becoming socially isolated in the event of a health condition or other major life change. Make sure you don't take these relationships for granted and that you continue to make them a priority in your life.

Secret #8: Build Your Resilience

Being resilient means that you are able to adjust easily to change. Throughout this book we've talked about how having a positive attitude, eating a good diet, and engaging in physical activity can help build your resilience to illness or mental decline. Maintaining a solid social support network can also help you roll with life's punches.

Studies show that older adults with good social support networks have a lower risk of becoming physically ill, a lower risk of depression and cognitive impairment, and an overall lower risk of death. Having good social support may also help you get better medical care. One study of Medicare beneficiaries revealed that only about four out of ten are accompanied by a friend or family member to medical appointments. Companions of these beneficiaries helped to ask questions, make comments, and write down information, like doctors' instructions. Beneficiaries with a companion's support reported being happier with their overall medical care and physician communication than those who were unaccompanied.

Your social network can consist of anyone—your spouse, children, grandchildren, friends, neighbors, and even clergy or medical professionals who care for you. Strive for six social contacts each month among the members of your network. That may sound like a lot, but what counts as a social contact does not have to be a formal, hours-long activity. Even a brief conversation with a friend counts—in person is best, but telephone contacts count, too. And you can combine contacts—going to church and then having lunch with friends afterward count as two social contacts.

Friends and Family Make Life Better Than Ever

Joyce is a sixty-one-year-old single working mother and grandmother. Her very busy schedule made her quite fatigued and unable to do much formal socializing.

When Joyce was diagnosed with breast cancer five years ago, she was stunned. She underwent surgery and subsequent medical treatments but often felt like giving up. Her friends and family, however, rallied around her and jumped in to help. She eventually felt well enough to join a breast cancer survivor group, where she formed some close friendships. Joyce is now cancer free and more active than when she was younger. She walks or bikes every weekend with her friends. More important, she feels able to tackle any life challenge because of her strong support network.

Support Your Mind and Your Social Network

Supporting your mind means stimulating it to stay sharp while preventing social isolation and mental health problems like depression. Stimulating your mind (especially with interactive activities) and maintaining a good social network go hand in hand. The best way to start this mutually beneficial relationship is to get involved.

Any activity will suffice, but research shows that some activities in particular, like acting, painting, and other artistic endeavors, photography, dancing in groups or with a partner, and doing volunteer work, benefit both your brain and body. Consider mentoring a child in your community who doesn't receive enough one-on-one attention. Your wisdom and time will be invaluable to that child and in return it will help keep you young.

Participating in social activities helps stimulate your brain to release "feel-good" chemicals like norepinephrine, which leads to feelings of happiness and contentment. In addition, when you are engaging in social relationships, an area of your brain called the posterior superior temporal sulcus gets an added workout. This same brain region is thought to be responsible for altruistic behavior.

Work for a Purpose

Exercise your altruism by giving back to others or your community. You can do it on a small scale (volunteering for simple tasks) or on a larger scale (setting up a social capital network in your area).

Consider a second career to enhance your social network. A group called Encore.org serves a growing network of people who want the personal fulfillment of giving back, along with continued income. Encore.org provides resources and connections for individuals and organizations establishing "encore careers" that combine social contribution, personal meaning, and financial security.

With your lifetime of knowledge, experience, and talent, you may have formed ideas about how to solve some of society's pervasive problems. Putting your ideas into action could make you eligible for a Purpose Prize. The Purpose Prize recognizes outstanding achievements by awarding investments of up to $100,000 and helps to create a network of people wanting to use their retirement years for the greater good. Since 2006, many over-sixty social innovators have been awarded this prize to help them with their endeavors. Some of them are:

Robert Chambers, age sixty-three: A former used-car salesman, Mr. Chambers was unhappy with the way dealerships would often prey on low-income buyers, who desperately needed reliable transportation to keep their jobs and care for their families. He formed Bonnie CLAC (Car Loans and Counseling) in his native New Hampshire to help low-income families receive low-interest loans to buy fuel-efficient cars.

Sharon Rohrbach, age sixty-five: During her sixteen-year career as a neonatal nurse in St. Louis, Ms. Rohrbach watched many newborn babies leave the hospital, only to return soon after with life-threatening conditions. She founded the Nurses for Newborns Foundation—a low-cost, high-impact program that sends experienced nurses to the homes of high-risk babies to provide skilled care, parental education, emotional support, and basic supplies.

Gary Maxworthy, age seventy: After a thirty-year career in the food distribution industry, Mr. Maxworthy was keenly aware that although there is no lack of fruit and vegetable farms in California, fresh produce rarely gets to those who use the state's food banks, where there is a preponderance of processed foods. He started an initiative called Farm to Family, which now distributes millions of pounds of fresh fruits and vegetables to food banks in California.

Information about the purpose prize can be found at www.purposeprize.org.

If you're feeling especially adventurous, the Peace Corps might be a good fit. Traditionally geared toward younger volunteers, the Peace Corps has been recruiting more seniors after seeing a spike in interest. The organization has also made many adjustments to accommodate older volunteers, including emphasizing oral and visual teaching, making it easier to learn languages, and stocking offices with medications for age 50-plus maladies.

A Late Blooming Technology Whiz

Caroline is a seventy-six-year-old grandmother who regularly babysits her two grandchildren on weekday afternoons. She considers herself a social person who likes to try new things but has always been a little intimidated by emerging computer technology. She's amazed at how easily her grandchildren adapt to complex video games and computers.

When the Nintendo Wii system first came to her Erickson community, she was reluctant to join in at first but gradually became active in nationwide Wii bowling tournaments. Soon after that, she was selected to try some new technology-driven brain exercise programs. Caroline found that she had a knack for the games and decided to take some on-campus computer classes. Now she's considered the expert among her friends when it comes to any technology, and word has spread. She's met scores of new people and frequently helps other Erickson residents who are hesitant to try new technologies.

Go Beyond Your Safety Zone

Don't be afraid to try new things. When you decide to be more involved with your family, friends, or community, it may be tempting to only participate in familiar activities. Remember: You don't want your brain to become hardwired and your routines predictable and boring.

Would you be willing to try something outrageous? What if it were for a good cause? It may be one of the best ways to keep what you've got.

A group of women at one Erickson community, Greenspring, did just that, with their Greenspring Calendar Girls initiative. This group of friends wanted a new way to raise money for residents who needed financial help. One evening, after a few glasses of wine, they came up with the idea of a racy calendar featuring . . . themselves. They set up scenarios, arranged to be photographed, and finally produced the type of calendar more typically sold on college campuses. These "calendar girls," however, were grandmothers and great-grandmothers ages sixty-nine to ninety-two.

The Greenspring Calendar Girls were an instant sensation. They were featured on the front page of Yahoo's Web site as well as national news venues. They sold so many calendars that their families were proudly embarrassed. According to Marguerite, one of the Greenspring Calendar Girls, "When my son saw my picture—posing with a guitar as if I had no clothes on—he said, 'Mother! Didn't you have anything better to do?' But I think he liked the calendar because he bought several!"

The success of the calendars (tens of thousands of dollars raised for residents in financial need) gave men at Greenspring the desire to do their own calendar—and the "Hunks of Greenspring" calendar was published for 2009, benefiting the same cause. All participants, including models, set designers, photographers, and makeup artists, were recruited from Greenspring residents and staff.

A simple idea hatched by a small group of friends in one woman's living room became a way for everyone involved to expand their social networks. New friendships have been made, and hundreds of people in the community have become involved. It helps everyone—those who need the additional financial support, and those who experience the thrill of being involved in their community, stretching their comfort zones, and meeting new people.

Get Back What You Can

What can you do if you're not particularly satisfied with your social network and want to expand it? What if you've moved to a new community and want to meet more people? What if you are bored with retirement?

You don't need to look too far. You might already have an existing social network that you can build upon—like your family or a church, synagogue, or mosque group. Start by attending more family events or functions at your place of worship. Use the lifelong knowledge gained from your career and hobbies to volunteer in your community. Look up old friends and plan some fun activities with them. Join a club to learn something new—like how to golf or speak a foreign language. Your options are limitless; just be sure to choose something you'll enjoy.

Socialize with Your Furry Friends

Pets can provide the benefit of constant companionship for people who may not have family or friends close by, or who might not get out very much. One case study describes an eighty-nine-year-old widow with diabetes who lived alone and complained to her doctor that she felt nervous, anxious, and lonely. She asked for medication to combat those feelings.

After being evaluated by a physician and a psychiatrist, the woman was found to be experiencing social isolation. As defined by the National Academies' Institute of Medicine, social isolation is "the absence of social interactions, contacts, and relationships with family and

Finding a New Life after a Late Divorce

Charles is a sixty-seven-year-old who went through a difficult divorce soon after retiring. Wanting to make a new start, he moved to another state. Once he had settled in, however, Charles found himself without a social network. He only spoke to his family by telephone and gradually lost touch with most of his friends and acquaintances in his former state of residence.

Charles wanted to get out and meet new people, so he relied on what was familiar. He used his background as a pastor to earn extra money by presiding over weddings and funerals. He met a surprising number of new friends this way. Charles also had military experience, so he joined a veteran's group and attended social activities. At one dance, he met a wonderful woman named Abigail, whom he later married.

friends, with neighbors on an individual level, and with 'society at large' on a broader level."

The woman's doctor contacted an animal shelter, and the woman received two kittens. She started to refer to them as her new family. As a result, the woman said she felt less anxious and fearful, and she also had better control over her diabetes.

Pets are not only constant companions for you, they can also help you meet new people. Take your dog out for walks in your community or the local dog park. Social clubs are available for people with almost any kind of indoor-only pet (check with your veterinarian or pet store). And if you love animals but don't want to own one, volunteer at a local pet shelter.

Compensate When Necessary

Many older adults find their social networks greatly diminished for two reasons: either the loss of a spouse or the onset of an illness or disability that's greatly affected their daily functioning. In either case, it's imperative for your good health that you stay connected.

Losing Your Spouse

Many surveys show that people rate the death of a spouse as the number one most difficult life event they've had to endure. Other research statistics illustrate the profound negative effects on the surviving spouse: Someone age forty-five to sixty-four who is grieving his/her spouse's death is 27 percent more likely to die than someone who has not recently lost a spouse. For people over age sixty-five, one study showed that the death of a wife in the past thirty days increases her husband's risk of death by 53 percent, and a husband's passing increases his wife's risk of death by 61 percent.

Regarding social networks, many men are more adversely affected by a wife's death because very often the wife was responsible for maintaining the couple's social calendar. In addition, some men live vicariously through their wives' social activities. Women, on the other hand, tend to suffer more financially when their husbands die, and a lack of money can greatly affect their ability to get out and socialize.

Grief is a normal reaction to a painful loss. The first phase of grief usually lasts up to two months. Some milder symptoms may last for a year or longer. If you have lost your spouse, you may have crying spells, appetite changes, and difficulty sleeping. Grief should not be denied because it is a healthy response to loss, but if you experience any of the following, call your doctor:

- You are overwhelmed by grief.

- You are using excessive amounts of drugs or alcohol.

- You become very depressed (sleeplessness, difficulty eating, apathy).

- You have prolonged depression that interferes with your daily life.

Getting additional support from clergy or support groups may help you deal with grief. Most important, stay engaged with friends and family who will want to help—let them. Resources are listed in Appendix A.

A Centenarian's Perspective

Anne is 101 years old. She met her husband Chester in high school, and they were married for nearly seventy years before he passed away. Anne had a long career as a pediatrician and had been through many triumphs and tragedies with her patients, as well as plenty of ups and downs in her own life. Although she was not affected financially by Chester's passing, his death was the most difficult and significant event of her long life.

Anne was fortunate enough, however, to have a few close friends to lean on. She talked with them about her loss, and they, in turn, shared their stories with her. This helped Anne to feel less isolated and eased her transitions through the grieving process.

A Gradual Adjustment after the Loss of His Wife

Not long after his children had grown and moved away, Thomas, now an eighty-two-year-old retiree, lost his wife. Thomas was not fond of showing his feelings, so he grieved for her mostly in isolation. Gradually, he talked to his family less often and stopped seeing friends.

After some time, Thomas realized how isolated he'd become but feared reestablishing social contacts because he felt like the only one who wasn't part of a couple. To overcome his fear, he started accepting his former golf buddies' invitations, which were men-only outings. He went to a few support-group meetings for people who had lost spouses, where he learned that his feelings were normal. He started going out with others from the group, and this contact gave him the confidence to become reconnected with his family and old friends.

Thomas still misses his wife but feels like he has gradually adjusted to a new life without her.

Secret #9: Seek Help

Seeking and accepting help for your health care needs, home maintenance, transportation, and so on does not mean that you are losing your independence. As you age, don't expect that you'll be able to do everything yourself. Trying to keep up like you used to in light of a changing health status or loss of family support can be detrimental to your physical health and interfere with what you need to do for your mental and social well-being. Plus, having additional support from others will provide more social interaction with the outside world.

More Peace of Mind without Her Car

Giving up your car can be a big blow to your sense of self-sufficiency and independence. But in some cases, relinquishing your car keys forever might be a good move—both for your overall health and financial security.

Hannah is a seventy-two-year-old former educator. She had always owned her own car, and her current one was paid off. Hannah drove her car two or three times a week, usually for shopping, church, or other errands. Her family members often drove her for family gatherings, and a family member or friend usually took her to medical appointments. Hannah's vision wasn't as keen as it used to be, and she found herself increasingly anxious each time she drove herself anywhere.

Although she didn't have car payments anymore, Hannah calculated how much the car cost her each year in gas, insurance, maintenance, repairs, tags, registration, and emissions testing. She compared those costs with the costs of a taxi service a few times a week. The taxi service turned out to be significantly less expensive than owning her car. In addition, Hannah no longer had to worry about the hassles of traffic or parking. Her financial savings meant more freedom—she now had extra funds to spend on social activities and found that she was busier and happier than ever.

Find the Help You Need

Your retirement years are the time to seek help so that you can free yourself and participate in a richer, more socially active life. Whether it's help with household tasks, bills, or transportation, your doctor is an excellent resource. Your doctor can work with a social worker, who can help you identify your needs and local resources for getting those needs met. You can also check your place of worship, as most are in touch with the most helpful community resources. Appendix A lists some national resources.

Test Your Social Health

This is a test that measures your level of social engagement, adapted from research conducted by British gerontologist Kevin Morgan and his colleagues.

Answer Yes or No to the following questions:
1. Do you read a newspaper or magazine on a regular basis?
2. Did you vote in the last election (local or national)?
3. Do you attend religious services or events?
4. Have you had a personal telephone conversation in the past week or so?
7. Do you browse or read books and materials from a library or bookstore?
5. Have you read or written a personal note (letter or e-mail) in the past week or so?
6. Have you attended a meeting or event of a club, group, or society in the past month?
7. Do you have a reliable mode of transportation to go shopping?
8. Do you have a full-time, part-time, or volunteer job?
9. Have you been away for a vacation in the past year or so?
10. Are you planning to go on a vacation in the next year or so?
11. Do you interact with friends/family as much as you would like?
12. Do you have at least one friend or family member living within easy driving distance?

13. Can you leave your home and walk independently out-side (with or without a cane or walker)?
14. Do you get out and do things as often as you would like?
15. Do you have at least one friend or neighbor that you could ask for urgent help if needed?

Give yourself one point for each Yes answer.
Scoring:
13–15: Your social health is excellent.
10–12: Your social health is fair.
9 or fewer: You need to work on improving your social network.

Social Networks at Work

Working past age sixty-five, whether full- or part-time, is becoming increasingly popular among today's older adults. Approximately two-thirds of AARP members work, and having a workplace is one of the easiest ways to augment your social network. A Gallup study found that people with at least three close friends at work were 96 percent more likely to be extremely satisfied with their lives. A 2006 study by Ameriprise Financial found that 40 percent of respondents (interviewed five years after retiring) reported that they were happier when they were working.

Always Invest in Your Social Life

Often we take our social lives for granted. We sometimes even take our friends and family for granted, that they will be there for us, but your social support network is like a bank account—the more you invest in your relationships, the more dividends and returns you'll enjoy.

We hope that in this chapter we've been able to explore some of the ways you can enhance your current relationships as well as some creative places to forge new friendships. By becoming more active in your community or in a specific work capacity, you not only naturally create new social networks that strengthen your life, you might also find yourself getting some unexpected physical and mental workouts. If by chance your work or activity pays you for your time, it can also benefit you financially, which we will discuss in the next chapter.

CHAPTER FIVE

Investing in Your Finances

"A nickel ain't worth a dime anymore."

—Yogi Berra

One of the biggest concerns for many older adults is running out of money. Products and services seem to cost more each year, yet many people live on fixed incomes. Although some retirement payments, such as from Social Security, are adjusted to try to account for inflation, many people believe these adjustments are inadequate, especially in the face of rapidly rising costs in health care, transportation, and other key areas of life. As a result, surveys show that two-thirds of Americans don't feel confident about having enough money for their retirement years and that money issues remain one of the top concerns that keep people awake at night.

Financial well-being is important because it allows you to invest in yourself—to eat well, stay active, and socialize—and to have the freedom to do what *you* want to do in life. Retirement can be expensive, and you can no longer expect to rely on the government to help meet your basic needs, much less enable you to live well.

Keep What You've Got

Major life changes, even if they're positive, can cause stress. Things that can make retirement stressful include changes in:

- income and financial status

- daily routine

- marriage or other family relationships and friendships

- health

Being stressed about money can be bad for your health. It can induce a vicious cycle—interfering with your sleep, eating habits, and overall mental well-being—potentially causing more health problems and costing you more in medical treatments.

Despite government estimates showing that a greater number of older adults have sufficient income to meet their basic living needs, many individuals still struggle with expenses, especially health care expenses. Some respond to their reduced circumstances by delaying or even foregoing medical treatments, and some cut back by reducing activities and social contacts, which can lead to isolation and depression.

Have a Plan

The key to keeping what you've got is to have a plan. Less than half of Americans admit having a good financial plan for their retirement. Studies show that financial planning is one of the life activities that people put off for as long as possible—or never get to. Perhaps it seems like a daunting and overwhelming task. But it doesn't have to be that way. Besides, why spend time worrying when you could be enjoying life knowing that you are financially prepared for your freedom years?

Developing a solid financial plan can be as simple as noting what you will do financially at major junctions in your life. The most basic financial plan should tell you how much money you'll need for retirement and where that money will come from.

Because your finances are as individual as you are, and just as no two people have the same medical profile or perspectives on how to manage their money, we can't lay out an individualized plan for you. We can, however, give you some direction about how to get one. The best way is to ask family or friends to recommend a reputable certified financial planner. Anyone can call themselves a "financial planner," but a *certified* financial planner (CFP) is someone who has passed a series of examinations and is trained to develop, implement, and coordinate your financial plan or formula. Research shows that most financial planning formulas calculate a higher level of financial need than what will in fact be necessary. But too much is always better than not enough, and the fees you have to pay for these services are well worth it in the long run. A certified financial planner gets paid in one of two ways: charging a consultation fee, or no fee and a commission on your investment choices, purchases, and sales. Always ask about the fee structure in advance.

In the absence of any personal recommendations, there are other resources you can use to find a certified financial planner, like the National Association of Personal Financial Advisors (www.napfa.org). Go to Appendix A for a list of government and private organizations.

Good Investment Advice in an Unstable Economy

When in late 2008 the housing and financial industries took a major hit, with stocks dropping to relative lows not seen since 1929, many of the hardest hit were retirees. Harvey, age seventy-two, recounts how he and his wife dealt with the situation: "We had a financial planner for years and were already living off of our retirement savings. When the stock market plunged, we met with our financial planner, who told us that our savings were down by about 25 percent. We were lucky, however, as many of our friends lost up to 40 percent of their investments. We didn't lose as much because at the very beginning of the economic downturn, our financial planner suggested that we convert some of our stocks to liquid investments. We're happy we took his advice, and we have been able to live a lifestyle that we are used to. Our friends, on the other hand, had to make adjustments because they had less money to spend in retirement. We count ourselves lucky to have had a good financial planner."

Retiring Early with the Help of Good Financial Planning

Edward and Evelyn, ages sixty-five and sixty-seven, got married later in life and shared the dream of an early retirement, during which they could enjoy their mutual interests and hobbies—travel, movies, fine wine, cards, and softball. They knew they needed a solid financial plan to achieve their goal, so they asked friends to recommend a good financial planner.

The planner they selected helped Edward and Evelyn formulate a plan, including participating in their *employers' matching retirement plans and investing a certain amount every month (over a number of years) in a diverse mix of mutual funds. As a result, Edward and Evelyn were able to retire in their fifties and now pack their days with friends and favorite activities.*

Retiring to Senior Housing

Gary and Elizabeth, ages seventy-five and seventy-two, married for fifty years, decided to sell their large house and move into a continuing care retirement community where they could enjoy an active social life and have access to dining, activities, and a maintenance-free environment. They used proceeds from the sale of their house to buy into the community and put the remainder in savings and investments. Best of all, they feel like they have an insurance policy on their finances: They no longer pay for utilities, property taxes, and other expenses that varied from year to year. Having avoided the surprises and pitfalls of managing an older home by themselves, they also know what their monthly expenses will be, and they feel like they have a home for life because their new community is a nonprofit organization that promises not to kick them out for an inability to pay. Gary and Elizabeth now fill their days with new and old friends, traveling, computer clubs, volunteering, and a diverse group of other interesting activities.

Get the Most out of Your Social Security Benefits

Most people envision retirement as a point in their lives where they stop working and start collecting Social Security benefits. In fact, continuing to work past the typical retirement age of sixty-two can enable you to maximize your Social Security benefits.

If no changes are made to the current Social Security system, benefits may decrease by 30 percent or more by the year 2041 or even earlier. The 2008 Retirement Confidence Survey showed that up to 45 percent of Americans age fifty-five and over expect Social Security to be a major source of their retirement income. Even if you won't be counting on Social Security as a major portion of your income, you still need to know how to get the most out of it. Here are some guidelines.

Wait to collect. Waiting to collect Social Security benefits can mean more money in your pocket for a longer period. If you were born January 2, 1942, through January 1, 1943, your age for full retirement benefits is sixty-five years and ten months. If you were born January 2, 1943, through January 1, 1955, your age for full benefits is sixty-six. If you work until your full retirement age or older, you may keep all of your benefits, no matter how much you earn. If you are younger than full retirement age, you can still collect benefits, but there is a limit to how much you can earn.

Apply three months before you need benefits. Social Security benefits don't start automatically. You will need your Social Security card, birth certificate, and your W-2 or tax forms from the previous year. Check with your local Social Security office for regulation changes or any additional required documentation.

Apply promptly for survivor's benefits if your spouse dies. Social Security benefits are not paid retroactively, and the sooner you apply, the sooner you'll receive benefits. There is also a small Social Security death benefit to assist with burial expenses.

Keep your information current. The Social Security Administration needs to know right away if you change your name or address. Not notifying the agency can cause a delay in payments.

Know your rights. Each year you receive an update in the mail from Social Security detailing your benefit eligibility. When you apply for benefits, the counselor will review this with you. If you don't agree with your benefit amount, you can contest it by contacting the Social Security Administration (800-772-1213 or www.ssa.gov).

Maximizing Income While Keeping Her Brain Sharp

Janice is a sixty-four-year-old marketing executive. She could retire at age sixty-six and still receive full Social Security benefits but has no intention of doing so. Janice explains: "I am a human being, not an age. I intend to keep working because then I can continue to receive a full salary as well as Social Security benefits. Working allows me to keep my mental capacities honed, keeps me active and engaged, and the extra money will enable me to keep spoiling my grandchildren!"

Secret #10: Put Your Money Where It Counts

Everyone's financial picture is different so the same financial plan will not work for everyone. But when it comes to protecting your nest egg, there are some tried-and-true strategies that make sense for just about everyone.

Be knowledgeable about your finances. Know how much you have in your accounts (including investments) and how well your money meets your risk profile. A financial advisor can be especially beneficial in helping you to determine this. And be prepared: Whichever spouse usually handles the household finances should teach the other how to manage them so that nobody is caught untrained in case of an emergency situation.

Protect your home's equity. If possible, avoid delving into your home's equity for minor renovations that do not add to the value of your house or for non-house purchases such as a boat or car.

Have both savings and diversified investments. Once again, your financial planner can help you determine what's best, but having a mixture of savings, stocks, bonds, money market accounts, and so on is usually a prudent move for your future financial security.

Pay off revolving debt monthly. If this isn't possible, pay off the highest-interest debts first. You can also negotiate credit card interest rates directly with your credit card company and may be able to lower these monthly payments by transferring debt to another lower interest credit card.

Keep six months or more of income saved at all times. Saving for those rainy days will help you handle unexpected medical or home repair expenses.

The Importance of Knowing Your Financial Information

Shirley and Charlie were married for over fifty years and raised three children together. Charlie had always taken care of the family's finances, but a few years ago, the family noticed that he was starting to become forgetful. He was subsequently diagnosed with Alzheimer's disease, and Shirley had to take over the finances.

Doing the monthly bills and keeping track of their savings and retirement accounts has made Shirley feel *anxious and stressed. Along with caring for Charlie, the extra burden of unfamiliar money management is sometimes overwhelming. Shirley, however, is fortunate that their daughter has been helping to manage their finances, but she regrets not learning how to manage them herself before Charlie's health declined.*

What You Need to Know about Your Household Finances

You need to know more than simply how to pay the bills each month. The more details you have about your finances, the easier it is to manage them. Even if someone else—a son/daughter or financial planner—is helping you with some items such as investments, you should know how to gain access to your financial resources.

Know where important financial papers are stored and have an organized system for maintaining your records.

Know what money you have in which accounts, like checking and savings accounts, certificates of deposit, retirement accounts, and other investments—stocks, bonds, or mutual funds.

Know details like bank/company names, account numbers, access numbers, login names, and passwords. Keep a key-accessible filing cabinet with this information, categorized by type of account (checking, savings, stocks, etc.), and another copy of this information in a safe place, such as a bank safe deposit box.

Know the status of your property investments, like your home, rental properties, vacation properties, or land. Keep a copy of land or property deeds in a safe place, such as a fire-safe deposit box at home or in a bank deposit box.

Know your credit card status—which cards you have, interest rates, and balances. Write down the credit card numbers and lost-card phone numbers for each credit card and keep this information in a safe place.

Know when to pay which bills whether they're monthly, like utilities, credit cards, and mortgages, or yearly, like property taxes or insurance. If you pay bills by mail, find a date each month and each year that meets the deadline for all your bills, and sit down on that date to pay everything. If you pay bills online, you can add this monthly reminder to your calendar and log into all your accounts to pay once a month. If you opt for automatic payments (where your monthly payments are deducted automatically from your bank checking account), periodically spot check these deductions to make sure the correct amounts are being paid from your account. By being organized and paying your bills on time, you avoid paying late charges and financing fees, which can add up to hundreds of dollars each month.

What Doesn't Work

Just as some financial strategies make good sense, others can be detrimental to your financial health. Some examples:

Using investment funds as emergency money. Research shows that people more readily dip into their investments rather than their savings accounts for emergencies. Given bank savings rates of approximately 1 percent or less per year and average long-term investment returns at 6 to 8 percent per year, it is better to use your savings because your investment funds will earn more in the long run. In addition, a large tax burden may accompany the withdrawal of investment money. Some people do not realize that their 401k plans were not taxed when the money was invested; as a result, upon withdrawal, these funds are considered taxable income. Moreover, if you withdraw your 401k money before a certain age, there are tax penalties as well.

Ignoring your credit profile. Federal law entitles you to a free credit report annually from each of the three major consumer credit reporting agencies. Review your reports each year to check accuracy, detect fraud, and learn your credit score. Knowing your credit score puts you in a better bargaining position when it comes to securing loans. For your free credit reports, go to www.annualcreditreport .com or call (877) 322-8228. (Note: You may have to pay a small fee for the actual score, but if your credit report shows a good track record of paying your debts, then your score is likely to be high and you may not need to know your exact number.)

Using debt to buy everyday items. If you do not usually pay your credit card bill in its entirety each month, using credit cards to buy groceries, gas, or personal items can result in having to pay more for these items later. Credit card interest rates are notoriously high, so unless you can completely pay off your balances each month, buy your everyday items with cash or with a debit card linked to your bank accounts.

Investing: Where to Keep Your Money

Where you put your money is dependent on your individual circumstances. In this section we will give you some basic information about common investments that may help you plan for a better retirement.

Saving Your Money

There are many ways to save money. The following section lists some of the most common. Evaluate your personal needs and financial plan before deciding on the best way to save.

Traditional bank savings accounts tend to have the lowest interest rates but are also the most liquid. Make sure that your bank is Federal Deposit Insurance Corporation (FDIC) insured for your money's safety.

Online savings accounts usually have significantly higher interest rates than traditional bank savings accounts. Reputable ones are FDIC insured and make it easy to access your money by transferring it to a regular checking or savings account at your usual bank.

Certificates of deposit (CDs) offered by banks are FDIC insured and usually have higher interest rates than comparable investments. Your money, however, is tied up for anywhere from three months to six years, and there are penalties for early withdrawal.

U.S. Treasury options, including Treasury bills (short-term), Treasury notes (medium-term) and Treasury bonds (long-term—also called U.S. savings bonds) are considered very safe investments. Treasury bills bear no interest but are sold at a discount and grow to maturity within one year. Treasury notes have fixed interest rates that are paid semi-annually and mature between one and ten years. Treasury bonds also have interest that is paid semi-annually but mature at ten years or more.

Money market accounts are savings accounts that share some of the features of money market funds. They are FDIC insured and usually have higher interest rates than traditional savings accounts. Money market account funds are liquid, although the number of transactions allowed on them may be somewhat limited.

College savings accounts are a good way to save money for the specific purpose of educating your children or grandchildren. There are many types of plans available, including 529 plans, which are tax-advantaged savings programs administered by states to encourage saving for higher education, and education individual retirement accounts, now called Coverdell Education Savings Accounts. Coverdell contributions are not tax-deductible, but earnings grow tax-deferred until withdrawn. Money withdrawn prior to a child turning age thirty to pay for elementary, secondary, or postsecondary education expenses is not subject to federal income tax.

Other accounts for children or grandchildren, not necessarily for education, include accounts set up under the Uniform Gifts for Minors Act (UGMA). UGMA was enacted to provide a simple way to transfer cash gifts or securities to a minor without the complications of a formal trust. Similarly, the Uniform Transfers to Minors Act extends the definition of "gifts" to include real estate, paintings, royalties, and patents.

Using "Perks" and Incentives to Save Money

Arlene is a seventy-six-year-old woman who never married or had children. As a younger working woman, she dreamed of traveling extensively once she retired but knew she'd need a solid retirement plan to finance her plans.

As Arlene got older, she worked on her financial plan. She got advice from friends and family and based her plan mostly on savings and government bonds. She began to realize, however, that even in the best of circumstances she would need to live conservatively in order for her money to last. Because Arlene worked for a major airline, she decided to investigate employee perks. She discovered that she could travel quite cheaply without having to wait until retirement. Looking back, Arlene is happy that she was able to travel around the world before retiring. Now she feels more secure about her financial future and can still take an occasional trip.

Planning for Income during Retirement: Retirement Accounts

Company-sponsored pension plans have largely gone the way of the dinosaur. Those who are facing retirement today will need to have other options to ensure a steady income and a comfortable future.

Employer-sponsored retirement accounts. These can be traditional 401k or 403b plans with your employer matching a percentage of your contribution amount. Money is deducted before taxes, and you decide how to invest—choosing from options provided by your employer's investment manager. Studies have shown that most people leave their money invested in the default option and do not make changes to their plans' investment mixes. Take a more active approach: Consult with your financial planner to customize your investments for a mix that meets your specific retirement needs.

Individual retirement accounts. If you don't have a retirement account at work, you can set up an individual retirement account (IRA) at your bank or brokerage. Traditional IRAs are tax deferred until you withdraw the money, and Roth IRAs have taxes taken out prior to being deposited. Keogh plans are another type of IRA designed for small business owners and the self-employed.

Annuities. Annuities are contracts issued by life insurance companies that pay installments in exchange for an initial lump-sum investment that may accumulate in value. Annuities are complex products with various structures and payment plans and are generally ideal for long-term investing. Although annuity contracts are defined by the Internal Revenue Code and regulated by individual states, fraud can occur. Beware of commissioned salespeople or advisors who try to persuade you to change products.

Other Investments

Other common investments include individual stocks, mutual funds, and property. Because both the stock market and real estate market are so volatile, you should always seek advice about whether either option is ideal for you. Investing is a complicated subject, and how you invest is based on your individual needs, preferences, and financial status. In general, however, conventional wisdom holds that you should diversify your investments—have a combination of stocks, bonds, real estate, money market funds, and so on. A higher level of liquidity is more desirable the older you get.

Investing in Your Home

How do you view your home in relation to your life's financial plan? As an important investment or as a burden? If you own your home, it can be one of the best investments for your retirement years. Research shows, however, that older adults tend not to invest in their homes—ignoring or being unable to maintain the necessary repairs. Not keeping up with your home's maintenance can erode the value of this important asset. If your home is a burden, you can either sell it and move to a more suitable environment or make your home more accommodating to your aging process.

Many older adults want to age "in place," that is, continue to live in their homes independently, safely, and comfortably regardless of their age, changing health, or functional abilities. Making your home accommodate your changing needs can involve simple steps (relocating your bedroom to the first floor, reducing trip hazards, or installing better lighting) or more complex remodeling (installing grab bars or raising/lowering counters and cabinets). If you need professional help, the National Association of Home Builders has a Certified Aging-in-Place Specialist program

(CAPS). CAPS professionals include home remodelers, general contractors, designers, architects, and health care consultants who are trained to help older adults increase access and maneuverability in their current homes. For more information call the National Association of Home Builders at (800) 368-5242 ext. 8216 or visit www.nahb.org/caps.

Is an Intentional Community Right for You?

Intentional communities are a growing trend among Americans age fifty and over. These organized groups allow older adults to lead safe, healthy, productive lives in their own homes by organizing and delivering needed programs and services like home maintenance, cooking, cleaning, shopping, transportation, home health, and concierge services for a membership fee. Intentional communities are member-initiated and member-controlled. An example of a large and successful intentional community is Boston's Beacon Hill Village (www.beaconhillvillage.org).

All intentional communities are considered subsets of naturally occurring retirement communities (NORCs), where large concentrations of older adults live and can help one another get better rates for certain services, participate in activities, or do other things together because of their sheer numbers and proximity. NORCs are either informal or formal arrangements: Sometimes you might not even know that the area you've been living in has become a NORC—your neighborhood may have naturally aged, more older adults have moved in over time, or groups of your friends may have moved closer as they've aged. Most NORCs in the United States do not have Web sites, so it is best to ask around to see if your community is a NORC.

Insurance

Insurance is a system designed to protect people against the risks of financial loss by transferring those risks to a large group who share the financial losses. Having the right insurance can help you maintain your financial health. But what types of insurances are absolutely necessary for older adults? Good health insurance is vital: Visit two to three insurance brokers to see if you have the best plan for your needs. In addition, long-term care insurance and life insurance are important products to seriously consider.

Rising Health Care Costs

You are spending more than ever on health care. In the United States, more than half (55 percent) of total health care costs are paid for by private funds, including private health insurance and consumers' out-of-pocket spending. Public programs, including Medicare and Medicaid, pay for about 45 percent. Health care costs are rising faster than inflation, however, and out-of-pocket spending by Medicare beneficiaries is high and expected to keep rising. Older adults currently spend an average of 18 percent of their cash income on health care. This 18 percent includes out-of-pocket expenditures, Medicare premiums, and individually purchased supplemental insurance.

Your health care spending will be higher if you have more health conditions. Taking care of yourself and thus investing in your health by employing preventive health care practices as discussed in Chapter Two can save you a lot of money in both the short- and long-term.

About Medicare

We can't discuss your financial health without mentioning Medicare. By some projections, if no changes are made to the system, Medicare may not be solvent by 2019. Surveys show that today's retirees are less confident in the future value of Medicare benefits than in previous years.

The Medicare system is buckling under its own weight. Medicare works now because enough working people pay into the system. But an aging U.S. population means fewer workers and more Medicare beneficiaries. This worker-beneficiary discrepancy is expected to grow larger, with some projections showing that by the year 2030, there will be 200 percent more Medicare beneficiaries than today, but only 18 percent more workers paying into the system.

A Medicare Primer

What is Medicare?

Medicare is a health insurance program for people age sixty-five and older, some people with disabilities who are under the age of sixty-five, and people with end-stage kidney disease.

Medicare Part A covers hospitalization. There are no premiums for Part A if you are sixty-five or older and receive (or are eligible for) retirement benefits from Social Security or the Railroad Retirement Board. You also do not have to pay premiums if you or your spouse had Medicare-covered government employment. If you are under age sixty-five, you will not have to pay premiums if you received Social Security or Railroad Board disability benefits for twenty-four months or you have end-stage kidney disease and meet certain requirements.

Medicare Part B covers medical expenses. You are not required to sign up for Part B when you become eligible but might be charged a penalty if you decide to sign up later. The premium for Part B is based on your income.

(continued)

Supplemental Health Insurance

Once you turn sixty-five, you are eligible for Medicare. Medicare doesn't cover everything, however, so for your financial health, consider supplemental health insurance coverage.

Supplemental policies for Medicare, called Medigap policies, are health insurance products sold by private insurance companies to fill gaps in Medicare coverage. Medigap policies help pay your share (coinsurance, co-payments, or deductibles) of the costs of Medicare-covered services. Some

---

Medicare Part C includes Medicare Advantage Plans, like HMOs and PPOs. This option combines Part A and Part B. Private insurance companies approved by Medicare provide this coverage and determine the cost. There are many payment options under these plans (variable premiums and co-pays), and the health care coverage is usually more than traditional Medicare provides. Opting for a Part C plan can save many people money, depending on their health and the plan benefits.

Medicare Part D is the prescription drug coverage portion of Medicare. You pay a premium for this coverage in addition to Part B premiums. If you choose a Medicare Advantage Plan, Part D might be included.

Where and when should I enroll in Medicare?

You can enroll in Medicare at your local Social Security office three months before your sixty-fifth birthday. If you sign up for Social Security benefits, you will be enrolled in Medicare Parts A and B at the same time. Medicare enrollment period rules are strict, so sign up for Medicare even if you do not plan to sign up for Social Security benefits.

Medigap policies cover certain costs that are not covered by Medicare.

Medicare Advantage Plans

Medicare Advantage Plans (also called Medicare Part C) are health plan options approved by Medicare and run by private companies. These plans sometimes provide extra benefits that aren't included under Medicare, and some may save you money. Medicare Advantage Plans include Medicare Preferred Provider Organization (PPO) Plans (usually a larger network of covered physicians and hospitals), Medicare Health Maintenance Organization (HMO) Plans (usually a more restricted group of covered physicians and hospitals), Medicare Private Fee-for-Service Plans (PFFS), Medicare Special Needs Plans (SNPs) (for certain chronic conditions such as chronic obstructive pulmonary disease [COPD] and diabetes, among others) and Medicare Medical Savings Account (MSA) Plans (combining a high-deductible health plan with a medical savings account—money that you put aside for health costs that beneficiaries can use to manage their health-care costs). See Appendix A for more information.

If you have a Medigap policy and are switching from original Medicare to a Medicare Advantage Plan, you no longer need your Medigap policy. Also, if you already have a Medicare Advantage Plan, it is illegal for anyone to sell you a Medigap policy unless you are changing back to original Medicare.

For more information about Medicare, Medicare supplemental policies, and Medicare Advantage plans, go to www.cms.hhs.gov/center/People.asp.

Handling Out-of-Control Health Care Costs

With health care costs rising, many older adults, especially those with several health conditions or even with only one serious condition, have to reconsider how to pay for necessary expenses without sacrificing quality care. Some ways to make changes include:

Make a detailed list of your monthly health expenses, including insurance premiums, co-payments, prescriptions, medical supplies, and so on.

Talk to several insurance brokers about which health insurance plans might be best for you based on your health expenses and medical needs. Some brokers are loyal to certain companies, so talking to more than one can give you a broader idea of your options.

Consider how a potential plan might cover you for unexpected circumstances—especially long hospital stays.

Investigate high-risk pools in your state. Up to thirty states now offer high-risk pools, which are government programs offering health insurance coverage to people who may be otherwise refused coverage by private insurance companies because of their health status. Although premiums may be high in these plans, it's better to have some coverage than none at all.

Look into health insurance plans provided by your trade, professional, or religious association. You may be eligible for special rates.

Long-Term Care Insurance

Studies show that many Americans do not know what "long-term care" services are, and most people do not know how much they cost. "Long-term care" is a catch-all phrase for services that meet both medical and nonmedical needs for people who can no longer care for themselves because of health conditions. For many people, long-term care is provided in nursing homes, where staff is present to help with needs such as eating, grooming, and medication management. (Many nursing homes also have short-term nursing care services for people in need of rehabilitation following surgery or other medical treatments.) Other people in need of long-term care can receive services at home, with family members and home care aides helping to take care of personal needs.

At the time of writing, long-term care in a nursing home costs, on average, over $100,000 per year. Unless personal assets have been depleted and the nursing home patient qualifies for Medicaid assistance, all of these costs are borne by the individual and/or the family. Long-term care at home is usually *more* expensive than nursing home care, generally costing over $120,000 per year. Again, these costs are usually borne by the individual and/or the family.

If the costs are not surprising enough, consider what percent of older adults will need long-term care services. People over sixty-five face a 40 percent risk of entering a nursing home in the future, and a majority of Americans will eventually need some form of long-term care. This need can quickly deplete carefully planned retirement and savings funds. What can you do to avoid this financial drain?

Long-term care insurance is a product that more and more Americans are buying after learning about the costs and odds involved in long-term care services. Only 5 percent of today's older adults live in nursing homes, but one of the biggest expenses in your retirement years can come when illness forces a loss of your functioning and you become dependent on home care or other long-term health care services.

Long-term care insurance helps pay for services not typically covered by Medicare or other insurance, such as nursing home care, assisted living services, adult day care, and home care services such as ongoing health monitoring by a visiting nurse or home health aide services. Many people don't think about long-term care until they get into their seventies and eighties. At these ages, however, you may be too high a risk for an insurer to cover you; or if you do qualify, the premiums may be prohibitively high. Because some long-term care policies have restrictions on age and health status, the best time to buy is in your mid-to late fifties, when you have the highest likelihood of being eligible for a policy and when premium costs might be lower.

Many people don't buy long-term care insurance because of misinformation—they think that Medicare or other insurances covers the costs. And studies have shown that people tend to ignore the possibility of low-probability, high-loss events that haven't occurred recently or that they think may never happen. It's simply human nature. But compared to other insurances like homeowner's and automobile insurance, the odds are fairly high that you will eventually need long-term care. Consider these insurance industry figures:

Odds of a fire in your home: 1 in 1,200

Odds of your car being totaled: 5 in 1,200

Odds of being hospitalized: 105 in 1,200

Odds of needing long-term care: 720 in 1,200

The bottom line: If you think you will be alive ten or more years from now, look into buying a good long-term care insurance policy.

What to look for in a long-term care policy

Policies can vary widely regarding coverage and other features. Look for the following in any policy you are considering.

At least one year of nursing home or home health care coverage, including intermediate and custodial care (care primarily for meeting personal needs such as assistance in bathing, dressing, eating, or taking medicine). Nursing home or home health care benefits *should not* be limited to skilled care (care ordered by a physician that requires the medical knowledge and technical training of a licensed health care professional).

Coverage for Alzheimer's disease or dementia, should the policyholder develop the condition after purchasing the policy.

An inflation protection option that includes a choice between automatically increasing the initial benefit level on an annual basis or a guaranteed right to increase benefit levels periodically without providing evidence of insurability.

An outline of coverage that systematically describes the policy's benefits, limitations, and exclusions, and also allows you to compare it with others.

A guarantee that the policy cannot be canceled, not renewed, or otherwise terminated because you get older or suffer deterioration in physical or mental health.

The right to return the policy within thirty days after you have purchased it and to receive a premium refund.

No requirement that policyholders either first be hospitalized or first receive skilled nursing home care in order to receive benefits.

Life Insurance

Many people regard life insurance as merely a way to pay for funeral expenses. But a good life insurance policy should cover much more, especially if you are responsible for caring for or supporting another person, or if you have financial obligations that would affect someone else if you die. Life insurance provides money for your beneficiaries for funeral costs, debts, estate taxes, future college tuition, or other current or anticipated expenses.

You can buy individual life insurance, or you may be able to purchase group coverage at a lower rate through your employer, professional association, union, or other organizations like AARP. Some life insurance policies ("whole life" policies) build cash values that you can use while you're still alive. Other policies ("term life" policies) do not build cash values and are therefore generally less expensive. Moreover, some policies require medical exams; those that don't usually have higher premiums.

The type of life insurance you purchase depends on your individual needs and the needs of your loved ones. For more information, see Appendix A.

Get Back What You Can

If despite your best estimates you think you'll still run out of money prematurely, make a new financial plan as soon as possible. Don't procrastinate. One study showed that although two-thirds of study participants thought their retirement savings were too low (and 35 percent said they planned to make changes), 86 percent had made no changes four months later. Procrastination tends to be the norm in retirement planning. For example, most retirement savings accounts allow you to reallocate funds to investments that you choose, but studies indicate that most people don't exercise this beneficial option.

Dealing with Debt

Some older adults face debt, whether it involves a mortgage, outstanding loans, or credit cards. Many debts are manageable as long as you preserve your income, but if your debts become unmanageable, here are some self-help tips:

Develop a budget. The first step toward taking control of your financial situation is to realistically assess how much you take in and how much you spend. Start by listing your income from all sources. Then, list your "fixed" expenses—those that are the same each month—such as mortgage payments, rent, car payments, and insurance premiums. Next, list your expenses that vary—entertainment, recreation or other activities, and clothing. Writing down all your expenses, even those that seem insignificant, is a helpful way to track your spending patterns, identify necessary expenses, and prioritize the rest. The goal is to make sure that you can make ends meet on the basic necessities: housing, food, health care, and insurance.

Your public library and bookstores have information about budgeting and money management techniques. In addition, computer software programs can be useful tools for developing and maintaining a budget, balancing your checkbook, and creating plans to save money and pay down your debt.

Contact your creditors. If you're having trouble making ends meet on your basic necessities, contact your creditors immediately. Tell them why it's difficult for you, and try to work out a modified payment plan that reduces your payments to a more manageable level. Don't wait until your accounts have been turned over to a debt collector. At that point, your creditors have given up on you.

Know your rights when dealing with debt collectors. The Fair Debt Collection Practices Act dictates how and when a debt collector may contact you. A debt collector may not call you before 8:00 a.m., after 9:00 p.m., or while you're at work if the collector knows that your employer doesn't approve of the calls. Collectors may not harass you, lie, or use unfair practices when they try to collect a debt. And they must honor a written request from you to stop further contact.

Focus on your automobile and home loans. If you stop making payments, lenders can repossess your car or foreclose on your house, and you lose valuable assets. Most automobile financing agreements allow your car to be repossessed without notice any time you're in default to the lender. If your car is repossessed, you may have to pay the balance due on the loan, as well as towing and storage costs, to get it back. If you see default approaching, you may be better off selling the car yourself and paying off the debt. You'll avoid the added costs of repossession and a negative entry on your credit report.

If you fall behind on your mortgage, contact your lender immediately to avoid foreclosure. Most lenders are willing to work with you if they believe you're acting in good faith and the situation is temporary. Some lenders may reduce or suspend your payments for a short time. When you resume regular payments, you may have to pay an additional amount toward the past due total. Other lenders may agree to change the terms of the mortgage by extending the repayment period to reduce the monthly debt. Ask whether additional fees would be assessed for these changes, and calculate how much they total in the long term.

If you and your lender cannot work out a plan, contact a housing counseling agency. Some agencies limit their counseling services to homeowners with Federal Housing Authority (FHA) mortgages, but many offer free help to any homeowner who's having trouble making mortgage payments. Call the local office of the Department of Housing and Urban Development or the housing authority in your state, county, or city for help in finding a legitimate housing counseling agency near you.

Consider a credit counseling organization. If you still can't keep track of your mounting bills, including credit card debt, bills for medical care, loans, and other debts, consider working with a credit counseling organization or service. These organizations serve consumers and their creditors by attempting to resolve debts using individualized debt repayment plans. The credit counseling service also seeks, when possible, a reduction in the amount of debt and a reduction or elimination of fees and charges accrued on the consumer's accounts.

Protect yourself by avoiding organizations that do any of the following:

- Charge high up-front or monthly fees for enrolling in credit counseling or a debt management plan (DMP).

- Pressure you to make "voluntary contributions," another name for fees.

- Won't send you free information about the services they provide without requiring you to give out personal financial information, such as credit card account numbers and balances.

- Try to enroll you in a DMP without spending time reviewing your financial situation.

- Offer to enroll you in a DMP without teaching you budgeting and money management skills.

- Demand that you make payments into a DMP before your creditors have accepted you into the program.

Reverse Mortgages—Worth It or Not?

Whether seeking money to finance a home improvement, pay off a current mortgage, supplement their retirement income, or pay for health care expenses, many older Americans are turning to "reverse" mortgages. These types of mortgages allow older homeowners to convert part of the equity in their homes into cash without having to sell their homes or take on additional monthly bills.

With a regular mortgage, you make monthly payments to the lender. But in a reverse mortgage, you receive money from the lender and generally don't have to pay it back for as long as you live in your home. Instead, the loan must be repaid when you die, sell your home, or no longer live there as your principal residence. Reverse mortgages can help homeowners who are house rich (but cash poor) stay in their homes and still meet their financial obligations.

To qualify for most reverse mortgages, you must be at least sixty-two and live in your home. The proceeds of a reverse mortgage (without other features, like an annuity) are generally tax-free, and many reverse mortgages have no income restrictions.

If considering a reverse mortgage, keep in mind the following:

- Lenders usually charge origination fees and other closing costs for a reverse mortgage. Lenders also may charge servicing fees during the term of the mortgage.

- The amount you owe on a reverse mortgage generally grows over time. Interest is charged on the outstanding balance and added to the amount you owe each month. That means your total debt increases over time as loan funds are advanced to you and interest accrues on the loan.

- Reverse mortgages may have fixed or variable rates. Most have variable rates that are tied to a financial index and will likely change according to market conditions.

- Reverse mortgages can use up all or some of the equity in your home, leaving fewer assets for you and your heirs. A "nonrecourse" clause, found in most reverse mortgages, prevents either you or your estate from owing more than the value of your home when the loan is repaid.

- Because you retain title to your home, you remain responsible for property taxes, insurance, utilities, fuel, maintenance, and other expenses. So if, for example, you don't pay property taxes or maintain homeowner's insurance, you risk the loan becoming due and payable.

- Interest on reverse mortgages is not deductible on income tax returns until the loan is paid off in part or whole.

There are different types of reverse mortgages, and if you are considering one, shop around to compare your options and the offered terms. Learn as much as you can about reverse mortgages before you talk to a counselor or lender. It will help you ask more informed questions, which could lead to a better deal. Be cautious if anyone tries to sell you something, like an annuity, and suggests that a reverse mortgage would be an easy way to pay for it. If you don't fully understand what they're selling, or you're not sure you need what they're selling, be even more skeptical.

Recently, there has been a trend of baby boomers (born between the years 1946–1964) taking reverse mortgages to purchase a treat for themselves—a boat, a fancy sportscar, or a new kitchen. If you consider your house an investment for the future and/or you feel like you do not have enough retirement savings, don't take a reverse mortgage to cover the costs of these types of purchases.

Compensate When Necessary

Catastrophic illness, death of a spouse, or other life events may put you in a position where you can't maintain your financial health without support. Even if you are able to work, you may need to rely on free or inexpensive resources to help you meet your basic needs for housing, food, utilities, transportation, or medical costs. See Appendix A for examples.

Cutting Back on Your Expenses

To effectively cut back, you need to know exactly where your money's going. Keep a notepad with you for a week or two and write down every penny you spend. Are there expenditures you could have avoided? If so, think about why you spent the unnecessary money and how you can avoid the same behavior in the future.

More ways to cut back:

- Destroy your credit cards. Pay down your debt and vow not to use borrowed money in the future.

- Evaluate your cable or satellite TV package to see if you can switch to a cheaper plan.

- Evaluate your telephone or cell phone package for cheaper plans.

- Get additional quotes for your car insurance. Switch if you can find a similar plan for less.

- Look for hidden fees at your bank. Change banks if necessary.

- Eat out less (includes carry-out) and cook at home more.

- Avoid brand-name foods when grocery shopping; choose store or generic brands.

- Cut, clip, and use coupons found in newspapers and magazines; many stores give you up to $1 off on items. Apply for your grocery store's special savings card—most major stores now offer special cards that offer in-store discounts when presented at check-out. Stores also send special offers and coupons to cardholders.

- Reduce your utility bills by unplugging infrequently used appliances, setting your thermostat to a comfortable level and not changing it, switching to energy-efficient lightbulbs, and contacting your local utility company to ask for a home inspection for potential energy wasters.

Cutting Expenses: What NOT to Do

Saving money does not mean sacrificing your health. If your health suffers, it may cost you even more in the long run. You can still maintain a healthy diet, exercise, and socialize, even with limited funds.

Don't forego fresh, homemade foods for seemingly cheaper canned and processed ones. Instead, look for sales on fresh fruits, vegetables, and bulk whole grains and meats. Look for stores that offer double or triple coupon savings. Plan your menus; freeze leftovers.

Don't stop exercising. Instead of paying for fitness center membership or exercise classes, go for walks with friends or exercise in your home with videos.

Don't isolate yourself. Instead of going out, invite friends over to watch a movie or to participate in neighborhood or community activities. Many local newspapers and municipalities publish a calendar of events on a week-to-week or monthly basis that often highlights low-cost but interesting community activities.

Making the Right Expense-Cutting Decisions

Gladys is seventy years old. She retired early several years ago because of medical problems (including diabetes and high blood pressure) and had little savings, relying mostly on Social Security and Medicare to get by. As her daily living expenses increased, she chose to cut back on groceries, often skipping meals and choosing the cheapest packaged foods, which were frequently high in salt, fat, and sugar. Soon her medical problems worsened, and Gladys found her medical costs rising because she needed more prescriptions, more diagnostic tests, and more doctors' visits.

Unhappy with her deteriorating health, Gladys made some other changes, like trading her cable television package for a less expensive one and giving up her weekly lunch with friends—instead suggesting they take turns hosting teas at their homes. She was able to save enough money to improve her diet and reverse some of the damage to her health.

Being Creatively Frugal

Anne is ninety-six years old and in fairly good health. She saved and invested carefully, but certainly never expected to live so long. Anne has always had a frugal side—she kept her old furniture and when traveling would often stay with friends—but as the years go by, she has learned even more ways to save money. She considers herself an accomplished user of food coupons and leftovers. She grows many of her own fresh vegetables and trades with friends and neighbors. She stays active by visiting friends for meals, going for walks, and cooking for others in her home. As a result, Anne's money has stretched to cover her unexpectedly long life, and she is content.

Finding a New Zest for Life After Losing It All

Robert and his wife Karen, ages sixty-four and sixty-three, worked hard for twelve years building a small media business and were able to sell it for a good profit. To enjoy their newfound retirement freedom, they consulted a financial advisor to manage their funds. He invested nearly all their money in the rapidly increasing stock market and then talked them into taking out a loan to purchase more stocks. When the 2008 global financial crisis occurred, Robert and Karen's investment portfolio suddenly collapsed. They also owed money on the loan.

For two months, Robert and Karen sat at home evaluating their stock portfolios and watching television news programs in disbelief and shock. After dinner with a friend, who raved about a Southeast Asian country he had just visited, Robert and Karen traveled to the same country and found themselves visiting the surrounding region on a shoestring budget. The travel helped to get their minds off their lost finances and enabled them to gain a new perspective on life. Traveling in Southeast Asia helped them save money, and a local international school offered Karen a job teaching. Since teaching was her former vocation before starting the business with Robert, Karen considered the offer. Because their three children were all grown and working, Robert could also relocate. Karen says, "When we lost our money, we thought, *What are we going to do? How will we survive?* But you know what? We'll be okay. It's still not good that we lost all that money, and we won't have the retirement we thought we would have, but it might actually be a better retirement in some ways. I think both of us have discovered a new way of living that is rewarding and enriching."

Using Your Support Network

Don't hesitate to rely on family, friends, or neighbors. Look for resources in your community or place of worship. In Chapter Two we talked about social capital groups—formal or informal community groups in which you can trade services among those in need in your neighborhood.

All communities differ regarding which resources are available. A good place to seek help is at your doctor's office. Your doctor is often knowledgeable about community resources and can also refer you to a social worker to help. Social workers can have many roles, but most are trained specialists in the social, emotional, and financial needs of patients and their families. Social workers can help you obtain needed services, like free or inexpensive meals, home modifications, home care, or help with medications or bills. Another good resource for public or nonprofit resources is your local or state office on aging.

To Work or Not

The definition of "retire" is to withdraw from one's occupation or conclude one's professional career. You may decide to give up your forty-hour work week and/or your professional career track, but working and retirement don't have to be mutually exclusive. You may want to work part-time to help pay the bills or receive certain benefits. Or there may be other reasons like maintaining your physical, mental, and social health.

Horace Deets, former executive director of AARP, interviewed several AARP members who lived to an advanced age and were still working. He found that many didn't necessarily need the extra money; they worked for a number of other positive and motivating reasons. One man said he had no choice but to work—it was ingrained in his "genetic code." Another said that his health would deteriorate if he stopped working. One ninety-year-old woman said she only needed two things in life—her vocation and an avocation—and that she felt at her best while engaging in both. In fact more than half the people surveyed said that not working was not included in their definition of retirement because they not only found the income helpful but also wanted a "more dynamic" lifestyle.

Today, retirement does not fit the traditional mold. In a 2006 survey ("New Retirement Mindscape" by Ameriprise Financial), 40 percent of people interviewed five years after retirement reported that they were happier when working.

Finding work

If you've been retired for a while and want to return to work, here are some suggestions.

Update your resumé. Besides your work history, include valuable life skills and knowledge that could translate into paid employment. Ask a friend who works in your preferred field to help review your resume and suggest changes.

Contact former employers. There may be part-time opportunities available. Your previous employers are aware of your good work history and can also serve as references for you.

Attend job fairs. Many local community centers and schools (such as your alma mater) host annual job fairs.

Bring a dozen copies of your resumé, and network with other people to see what is available in your area.

Investigate other avenues. At least half a dozen Web sites exist that are specifically designed for seniors' employment, like the Senior Job Bank (www.seniorjobbank.org). Other resources are listed in Appendix A.

Finding a job may take some time, but it's worth it for you to find a good fit—a company that values you and a job that you love. Maintain your sense of humor, and good luck!

A Fit Financial Future

You need money to stay fit in the other areas of your life, but very often financial constraints cause older adults to be overly frugal. While prudent spending is admirable, sometimes what you're *not* spending can backfire. Investing a little now in the right places can help you reap rewards later, and possibly change your retirement vision.

Learn more about how retirement is changing. People everywhere are looking for purpose, working part-time, volunteering, and remaining active. It's an exciting time to be living, and in Chapter Six, we'll show you how to get the most out of your retirement years.

CHAPTER SIX

Your Overall Retirement Vision

"It's not who's going to let me, it's who's going to stop me."

—Ayn Rand

Not long ago, people thought of retirement as an ending, a closing phase to life. Today, many people who reach their retirement years view this period as a new life chapter, filled with opportunities for growth and meaning. Some retirees refer to this chapter as "the bonus years," some as the "transitional" years. At Erickson, we call it "the freedom years."

The concept of retirement is completely changing. Since there are often several decades between typical retirement age and the end of life, society is just beginning to explore what this new life phase means. People retiring today are generally healthier and more financially secure than previous generations and therefore have more freedom to shape their retirements. In this section, we'll explore how to create a road map to your best retirement.

The Changing Concepts of Retirement

Your retirement is not your grandmother's retirement. Many retirees of your parents' and grandparents' generations lived on fixed incomes that included Social Security and/or partial pensions. Many experienced more complex chronic conditions, were not technologically proficient, and had limited independence. In fact, retirement for previous generations usually meant simply not working anymore. It was not viewed as an opportunity for positive life changes.

The traditional concept of retirement may have started in the late 1800s when the Baltimore and Ohio Railroad instituted a plan that made retirement at age sixty-five mandatory. This retirement plan also provided a pension for employees who had worked for the company for at least ten years—an incentive not designed to provide security or assistance to older workers but rather to discourage workers from changing jobs. At about the same time, labor unions proposed that seniority be the basis for layoffs and cutbacks, as the oldest workers tended to have the highest salaries. In addition to these changes, a significant influx of European immigrants started filling job vacancies at lower wages, and industrialization in the early 1900s meant a faster work pace and longer hours—both conditions that were better suited to younger workers. Older adult workers became increasingly viewed as obsolete.

By the 1940s and 1950s, the concept of retirement changed again as the older population doubled, partly due to medical advances. Many people had worked in war-related jobs with good pension plans. With the increasing availability of governmental assistance, retirement began to be viewed as a time of prepaid leisure, a reward for a lifetime of hard work. With increased financial security, more older adults were able to live independently instead of in the multigenerational households common to the past.

As we advance into the 2000s, we are seeing another change in what retirement means. Today's older adults as they prepare for their own retirements are healthy, technology savvy, and civically engaged. A 2003 AARP survey showed that seven out of ten older workers describe their retirement as having the following features:

- spending more time with family and friends

- receiving Social Security or pension benefits

- relaxing

- having more fun

- doing things they never had time for

The majority of respondents to this same AARP survey also said that their personal definition of retirement includes some form of work. A different study of fifty- to seventy-year-olds showed that almost 70 percent of those who had not yet retired planned to work into their retirement years or never retire, and nearly 50 percent planned to work past age seventy. While some of these older adults need to work past typical retirement ages because of financial constraints, studies also indicate that many people work because of the non-financial benefits of employment like personal enjoyment and social contacts.

Health and other personal problems may also influence who retires. Of those who retired between the ages of fifty and fifty-eight, one in four cited "health concerns" as very important in their decision to retire.

Older adults today expect fulfilling, interesting retirements. Although many look at retirement as a chance to pursue leisure interests, experience new things through travel, and spend time with friends and family, most retirees also want to be active in the community or in a work environment. At Erickson, we see more and more new retirees who continue work in some capacity.

Retirement Satisfaction

Despite societal views to the contrary, research shows that not all older adults are happy with the concept of retirement or satisfied with their transition into this new life phase. A 2006 study by Ameriprise Financial found that 40 percent of respondents (interviewed five years after retiring) reported that they had been happier when working.

Other researchers conducted a survey of retired people in Canada and discovered that approximately one-third of respondents had not adjusted well to retirement. The same researchers conducted a survey of over one hundred men several years after retiring and proposed that being bored, missing work relationships, and not adjusting to change had a more significant adverse impact on the participants than poor health or financial well-being.

The New Workforce

According to the U.S. Bureau of Labor Statistics, by 2010, 17 percent of the workforce will be made up of adults age fifty-five and older, up from 13 percent in the year 2000. At the same time, younger workers between the ages of twenty-five and fifty-four are expected to decline as a percentage of the workforce, from 71 percent in 2000 to 67 percent in 2010. Because the average age of the workforce is increasing, employers will need to recognize and address their aging employees' needs.

Ageism

Ageism is the untrue assumption that a person's chronological age determines their societal status and roles. It often manifests as a bias against older adults based solely on their age and can lead to discrimination in many aspects of life. Dr. Robert N. Butler, a gerontologist, first coined the term in the late 1960s when he was describing public resistance to senior housing.

We live every day with the perpetuation of pervasive stereotypes in print, movies, television, and advertising. Seventy-four-year-old Doris Roberts (who starred on the television series *Everybody Loves Raymond)* testified before Congress specifically on the topic of aging images in the media and noted that ageism is "the last bastion of bigotry."

When older adults of retirement age try to secure work, housing, or other services, many of them face age-related discrimination. The worst manifestation of ageism is when it results in abuse—physical, mental, and even financial— often the worst perpetrators being those entrusted with seniors' care.

Fighting Ageism

What is being done about ageism? The emerging demographic shift may help to change some negative stereotypes as older adults become more visible and influential in all aspects of American society. And there is legislation in place: The Age Discrimination Employment Act (ADEA), passed in 1967, made it illegal to fire, force to retire, or fail to hire workers strictly on the basis of age. But what can you do as one person to help combat ageism?

Keep thinking positively about yourself. Maintain a positive perspective about your aging process and your aging peers. Research shows that negative attitudes can affect longevity. One Yale University study revealed that older adults with more positive perceptions of aging lived seven and a half years longer than those with negative perceptions. The same researchers found that older people exposed to negative images of aging scored worse on memory and balance tests and showed higher stress levels.

Develop relationships with younger people. Dr. Bill Thomas, an international authority on geriatric medicine and eldercare and professor at the Erickson School of Aging Studies at the University of Maryland, says that strong relationships with young people make older adults less likely to hold ageist biases. Go beyond your family and get involved with children, adolescents, and younger adults in mutually rewarding activities like tutoring or mentoring.

Civic Involvement

Today's older adults seem to be equally or more civically engaged than previous generations. In one public policy and aging report, a researcher points to evidence that Americans ages fifty-five and over want to contribute "if the opportunities to do so are professionally planned, . . . flexible, meet a critical need, are meaningful, and leave a lasting impact." Another study shows that volunteer rates among people between the ages of forty-six and fifty-seven are much higher than those of previous generations.

Spotlight on Experience Corps

Experience Corps, an intergenerational program where adults age fifty-five and over tutor and mentor individual children in urban public schools, is one of the most well-researched civic programs in the United States for older adults. Founded as the brainchild of John Gardner, former Secretary of Health, Education, and Welfare, it began as a pilot project of the U.S. Corporation for National Service (the U.S. national volunteering and civic service umbrella organization).

Volunteers are grouped in teams of six to ten people and receive training in child development, conflict resolution, tutoring, and other helpful subjects. The schools selected for Experience Corps tend to be crowded urban schools where children may not receive as much individualized attention as they need. Volunteers primarily help children learn how to read or improve reading and writing skills.

Now implemented in over a dozen states, Experience Corps has been proven by a large team of Johns Hopkins researchers to be effective in improving the physical, mental, social, and financial health of older adults (as well as benefiting participating children and their families).

Hopkins researchers found that the Experience Corps program brings people out of their homes and makes them more physically active than before. Participants watched less television than nonparticipants over the course of one study. Forty-four percent of Experience Corps participants felt improvement in their physical strength compared with only 18 percent of nonparticipants. Moreover, those who participated in Experience Corps reported a 25 percent increase in the number of calories burned compared with 5 percent of nonparticipants.

Experience Corps also improves the mental abilities of volunteers, according to brain scans of participants versus nonparticipants (as described in Chapter Three). And although Experience Corps is a volunteer program, participants who serve fifteen or more hours a week receive a small stipend to help cover transportation costs as well as personal monthly expenses. The stipend is meant to encourage volunteers who give more time, but it does not preclude people who want to volunteer fewer than fifteen hours a week. A final testament to Experience Corps' effectiveness is that 98 percent of program participants reported being sat-isfied with their experiences in the schools, and 80 percent returned to participate again the following school year.

What started as a pilot project in the 1990s has blos-somed into a rapidly growing national program sponsored by major foundations and academic institutions. To see if there is an Experience Corps site near you or to find out more information about the program's impact, visit www. experiencecorps.org.

Today's Sandwich Generation

Many of today's older adults, especially those in the baby boom generation, are part of the sandwich generation—people who are "sandwiched" between their own growing family's needs and the needs of aging parents. At a time when they should be preparing for retirement, celebrating their children's accomplishments, and enjoying grandchil-dren, many are confronted with caring for parents in their eighties and nineties.

In a documentary called *The Sandwich Generation*, Julie Winokur and Ed Kashi estimate that up to twenty million American adults are caring for their parents in addition to being parents to their own children. The stress of this situ-ation can be overwhelming. Adult children often describe the feeling as simply trying to survive day to day because of conflicts and demands on their time. In addition, the aging parents are often frustrated by the fear of becoming a bur-den to their adult children.

Many resources can help those dealing with this situ-ation, including support agencies, private home care, and continuing care retirement communities with care avail-able for older adults at any level of independence. One of the most important resources is called respite care, where someone relieves the adult child temporarily from the care of aging parents. Web sites such as www.caring.com, www.caregiving.org, and www.familycaregiving101.org are also good places to find support. More helpful resources are listed in Appendix A.

Easing the Burden

James and Margaret, from Akron, Ohio, are both in their late fifties and have two children—one in college, and one who is married with two children of her own and living on the West Coast. Margaret's parents live in Massachusetts.

As an only child, Margaret solely carries the responsibility of caring for her parents, and the geographical distance compounded the problem especially when her mother had a stroke and her father was subsequently diagnosed with prostate cancer. After frequent exhausting trips, Margaret began exploring her options for ensuring quality care for her parents with the intent of moving them closer to her Ohio home.

Margaret and James visited several continuing care retirement communities before finally deciding on one that enabled her parents to be as independent as possible with on-site medical care, home support, and a wide variety of services and amenities. Her parents settled right in to their new community.

Margaret and James felt much better knowing that they could focus on their lives again while feeling assured that her parents were happy and well cared for. Margaret and James can now enjoy their children and grandchildren, continue with their own plans for retirement, and have the comfort of having her parents—their children's grandparents—close by.

Figure Out What Works for You

As you plan for retirement, keep in mind that what your friends are planning or what your family thinks you should do might not work for you. Everyone is different, and acknowledging these differences can make you happier and more satisfied with retirement when it's time for you to make the transition. For instance, would you find gardening at home boring or exciting? Would you find traveling exhausting or relaxing?

Friends Who Want Different Things

Barbara and Dick, ages seventy-three and seventy-two, raised six children together, which did not leave them much time or money to travel. Now that they are retired and their children are grown, Barbara and Dick love to go on cruises to places they have read about in books and magazines or have heard about from friends. Every year, they go on at least three cruises, either traveling to exotic places or visiting their children, who do not live nearby. They are sure, however, to be home for tax time: Dick was a former accountant and still prepares tax returns during the busy season for extra money. Barbara, on the other hand, is an accomplished baker and likes to bake cakes and cookies for charity bake sales during her time at home. And when not traveling, both also love spending time with their fourteen grandchildren.

Their friends Marguerite and George, ages seventy-three and seventy-six, spend their time quite differently. Because George was a manager for a large hotel chain, he took his wife and three children around the world while managing various properties. They lived in Bangkok, Amsterdam, Sydney, and many other cities. Marguerite and George also took the opportunity to travel to neighboring countries while they were in different locations. They therefore have seen a lot of the world and view their retirement as an opportunity to stay active while remaining close to home. They are involved with local political processes and help to sign up voters for local and state elections. They exercise every day, and Marguerite especially enjoys her weekly water aerobics class. These activities have enabled Marguerite and George to form a solid social network right in their own community.

It's Not Always Easy: The Unexpected

Ralph was a fifty-five-year-old steel worker looking forward to retiring at age sixty-five with a good pension and excellent retiree health benefits. Then the steel plant closed and the company folded, taking with it thousands of workers' salaries, pensions, and retirement benefits. Ralph was forced to find a new job that did not pay as well. He also had to make up for thirty years of lost retirement savings, which he knew would be next to impossible. Rather than despair, Ralph sought help from a local pro bono financial planning organization and decided to learn a new trade. He now has a new job as a plumber and is on track to retire according to his new personal financial plan.

While Ralph's new plan means he won't retire until age seventy, he does not feel down about it. In the course of creating his financial plan at the pro bono center, Ralph met a lot of other people who were in similar situations (or worse off) and that helped him maintain his positive perspective: He still has his health, a loving family, and a job that enables him to learn new things every day.

Who Is Ready for Retirement? (And Who Isn't?)

Research shows that at least half of baby boomers are prepared for a comfortable financial retirement. A significant number, however, are not, and this growing gap between the "haves" and "have-nots" could create a class of seniors that are more heavily dependent on both the government and younger generations. Other research shows that those who are single and/or have not graduated from high school are more likely to outlive their resources.

It is common to feel apprehensive about having a comfortable retirement, and among those who are prepared, many still have fears about financial security, their physical health, or broader fears about how they'll cope with such a major life change. Creating a retirement road map can give you peace of mind.

A Tale of Two New Retirees

David and Petra, ages sixty-four and sixty-two, sold their small travel business and looked forward to an enjoyable retirement. Petra tried to make up for lost time as a grandmother and doted on her young grandchildren, replacing her relationships with travel customers with those of her children and grandchildren.

David, however, grew depressed. He felt like he had lost his identity as a travel specialist as well as the relationships and interactions with his customers. Petra, knowing David's love of tennis, signed him up for a local tennis club.

At first, David refused to participate and resisted Petra's encouragement. Then one day, David decided to attend a youth tournament at the tennis club. He found himself signing up to help inner-city children learn and

> *improve their game. Soon things started turning around for David. He became happy and involved with life again because he had a new identity as a tennis mentor, new relationships with his mentees and their families, and a new passion for living.*

Prepare Now: Your Road Map to a Successful Retirement

What is your retirement vision? Do you see yourself working? Volunteering? Spending more time with family and friends? Traveling?

Many older adults have a vague idea about what they want to do after they retire, with no realistic plan in place. Conduct a thorough self-assessment in order to identify what's most important to you; then set achievable goals that will help you enjoy your retirement years to the fullest extent.

Consider Your Finances First

As we've emphasized throughout this book (especially in Chapter Five), money matters. Money helps you meet your basic needs and achieve your goals and objectives for optimal health, activities, independence, and long-term security. Have a solid financial plan in place and stick to it. Once you have a plan, you'll be better able to assess how much or how long you'll need to work before retiring.

Expenditures. Where will you spend your money after retirement? Experts claim that the average American will spend 70 to 90 percent of their current income to live a similar lifestyle in retirement. Studies show that those ages sixty-five to seventy-four spend 20 percent less than fifty-five to sixty-four-year-olds, and those seventy-five and up spend 30 percent less than those ages sixty-five to seventy-four. Your expenses may be more or less than those of someone else your age because of differing debts, health care expenses, recreational activities, etc.

Income. Where will your money come from after you retire? Some people receive a pension or defined benefit plan, which provides a steady income stream for life. Fifty-nine percent of workers surveyed expect to receive traditional pensions, but many people find that their pensions have been renegotiated by employers (with a reduction in benefits) and that future employers are not even offering pensions. Other people are relying heavily on Social Security, but it is best to plan on income from multiple sources, including retirement accounts, personal savings, home equity, and so forth. If you have money in stock or bond markets, it is critical to diversify your portfolio. In the event of a market downturn similar to the one in 2008, your retirement income stream will be more resilient.

Debt. Will you retire with or without debt? One in four retirees reports having debt levels equal to or more than their total income. Less than one in three reported having no debt at all. Carrying debt into your retirement years adds a level of stress that may negatively affect your health. It is important to take steps to reduce your debt (see Chapter Five).

Reduce Stress in Your Retirement

Although it may seem like an oxymoron, retirement can be stressful. Any major life change, even a positive one, can cause stress. Retirement, after all, means changes in your income status, daily routines, relationships with family and friends, roles and identity, and possibly your physical and psychological health. One Canadian study showed that one out of three individuals had not adjusted well to retirement. Another study found that being bored, not adjusting well to change, and not replacing lost work relationships had a greater negative impact on individual well-being than poor physical or financial health.

Depression is not uncommon among new retirees, and reports note that Caucasian men seem to have the hardest time adjusting to a retired lifestyle. Moreover, people who have had previous bouts of depression, who have marital problems, or who have a more pessimistic or hopeless life outlook are at greater risk of depression in retirement. If you are at risk for depression, talk to your doctor about what you can do now to prevent post-retirement depression. In addition, consider the following:

Your retirement process. Easing into retirement may be less stressful than abruptly stepping down from a full-time career. You could change to part-time work in your same career or work fewer hours in another capacity for your employer.

Your newfound leisure time. Identify what's most important to you and plan activities to match. Do you want to get more physically fit? Plan an exercise schedule. Do you want to stay socially connected? Work to maintain your current relationships with family and friends. Identify enjoyable activities where you're likely to meet new people with similar interests.

Having a list of goals can help you deal with unexpected stress. Follow these tips for creating a realistic goal list:

Make your goals achievable. If, for example, you want to be more physically fit, having a goal of "exercising every day" is not as achievable as "walk six days a week for ten minutes the first week, fifteen minutes the second week, twenty minutes the third week," and so on. A goal of "save money for emergencies" can be changed to "transfer (specific dollar amount) to savings/money market account on the first of each month."

Be flexible. When formulating or carrying out your goals, be flexible about changes. Economic factors, changes in your health or personal life, or other unknown factors may compel you to revamp your original plan. Make your retirement vision a "working document," one that you revise yearly or when you experience major life or priority changes.

Experiment. When implementing your goals, don't be afraid to try something new, especially if a particular goal isn't working out the way you planned. If you've made a wish list that details things you always wanted to do but never had time for, revisit it. Discover a new passion and pursue it.

Ask Yourself These Questions

When you formulate your goals, make them specific by answering the following questions:

What do I want to do? (Get a degree? Learn a new skill? Start a business?)

Who do I want to do it with?

When will I start?

Which necessary resources do I already have, and which do I need to find?

How can I make this goal happen?

Popular goals for retirees

Do you want the same things or have the same goals as you did twenty or thirty years ago? Not likely. Your goals may change frequently, and since you can plan on living a long time in this new life phase, write (and revise) your goals carefully.

It might seem difficult to start writing down retirement goals. But it doesn't have to be. Here are some goals that are popular with many new retirees.

Learn something new. Check your local community college, art league, or university for a selection of classes to take. Public libraries, community centers, and fitness centers also host a variety of classes. For topics of particular interest to you that may not be available in a class format, organize a book club or discussion cafe and invite friends.

Get Involved. Your local chapters of the Office on Aging as well as AARP have contacts for various volunteering opportunities and possibly also paid work. If you are an accountant, you might help disadvantaged families with their taxes. If you are a lawyer, you might help a widow with her legal needs. Public facilities such as museums and libraries are often looking for volunteers as well. One of the best places to volunteer your time and services is at a public school. Call around and see where you can put your skills to work.

See the world. If you are interested in other cultures and have the resources, check with a travel agent for pre-arranged tours to destinations that interest you. If you are more adventurous, go to the bookstore, find a travel guide, and arrange things yourself.

Retirement Readiness Quiz

Choose the answer that most accurately reflects your retirement plans.

1. Which statement most closely resembles how you think about retirement?
   a. I haven't had time to think about it.
   b. It will be like an extended vacation: mostly fun and leisure, when I will have time to do what I want.
   c. I will have time to pursue activities and interests that I haven't had much time for, and I plan to learn and experience some new things.

---

    d. It will be a balance of several activities and interests, which I can list now.

2. Who have you discussed your retirement plans with?
    a. I try to keep them to myself.
    b. My children and good friends only.
    c. My spouse or long-term partner only.
    d. My spouse/partner, children, and good friends.

3. What activities related to your work or specialty will you continue into retirement?
    a. None. I'm ready to be done with my work and look forward to relaxing.
    b. Not many because I'll want to try things that I've never done before.
    c. I will continue to work, then slowly transition by working less and adding other activities.
    d. I plan to volunteer with my skills, work part-time in my previous or a related career, or contribute to my profession in a meaningful way.

4. If you were away from work or your usual day-to-day activities for six months, what would you miss?
    a. Nothing.
    b. I'd be happy to miss all the stress and generally hectic lifestyle.
    c. My friends.
    d. Being part of an organization that has goals and a relationship-based environment.

5. What sorts of physical activity do you plan to have in retirement?
    a. I'd like to start exercising and lose some of the weight that I've put on.
    b. I do not exercise now, but I watch my weight carefully.

    c. I exercise once or twice a week and plan to keep it up;
I will also try to eat better.

    d. I exercise at least three times a week and watch what
I eat; I will probably keep this up into retirement.

6. How are you estimating the costs of your retirement
lifestyle?

    a. I've been too busy or too worried to think about it.

    b. I made some rough estimates of my retirement costs
but need to be more detailed about them.

    c. I believe it will cost approximately the same or a lit-
tle less than what I spend today; if I travel more, the
costs may be a bit more.

    d. I've made a fairly detailed budget of housing, food,
transportation, health care, travel, entertainment,
and other costs.

7. What are your health coverage plans in retirement?

    a. I will not have health insurance after I retire, so I will
have to save wisely to pay medical expenses.

    b. I will have coverage through work or through my
own policy before age 65, at which time I'll get coverage through Medicare.

    c. I will have coverage through work or through my
own policy before age 65, at which time I'll get Medicare and a Medigap policy.

8. In what order will you use your assets in retirement?

    a. I don't know or haven't thought about it.

    b. I'll use my retirement accounts first, then my per-
sonal/bank savings accounts.

    c. I'll use a portion from each of my capital sources
(Social Security, pension or retirement accounts, savings accounts, home equity, etc.)

    d. I have a plan on how to move my assets around and
what to spend given the taxation of each type of asset.

9. How have you estimated how much you will need for the rest of your life (and that of your spouse/partner)?
   a. I haven't had the time to do these estimates.
   b. I know on average how much longer someone my age (and that of my spouse/partner) lives and have used this information to calculate needs.
   c. I spoke with a financial or insurance planner about my personal profile and will use the information I received to make my cost estimations.
   d. I calculated my retirement financial needs; then I planned my future insurance and investment strategy as well as my retirement budget accordingly.
10. What will be the legacy you leave behind?
   a. I can't say what others will remember me for. Hopefully positive things.
   b. I have drafted a will that leaves my valuables and assets to loved ones.
   c. I want to do things now and in my retirement that people will remember me for.
   d. Future generations will remember me for the assets and values that I leave behind; specifically, I have done the following . . . (name ways).

Scoring

Give yourself 1 point for an "a" answer, 2 points for a "b" answer, 3 points for a "c" answer, and 4 points for a "d" answer. Add up your scores for the ten questions.

If you scored 35–39, you are ready (or very nearly ready) for retirement—financially, physically, socially, and mentally. Keep up the good planning.

If you scored 20–34, you are not quite ready for retirement—but almost. You might be missing some plans in one or more of the four areas: financial, physical, social, or mental. Look to see where your scores were low, and spend time planning what you want in these areas.

If you scored 10–19, you need to put some more time and thought into your retirement. Seek the help of a financial planner or life counselor to get yourself started.

How Young Will You Feel?

A study by the University of Michigan revealed that today's seniors feel, on average, thirteen years younger than their chronological age. The study ran for six years, and as participants aged, they felt closer to their actual age if they were in poor or declining health. Related findings conducted by the same researchers revealed that a positive attitude about aging was associated with improved health and longevity.

These research findings support Erickson's theories about aging, and why we say that old is the new young. If you maintain your health in all critical areas of your life you will feel younger. It all ties back to Secret #1: It can be done. The secret to adding life to your years is you. We've given you quite a lot of information in this book, but that doesn't mean you have to use all of it—after doing your self-assessments you'll know on which areas to focus. You have control when you make the right choices. It takes some work, but once you start making positive changes, you'll see improvements right away, and the journey to your best retirement will be realized.

"We can change the way we age by staying active, to the fullest extent possible, within all areas of life: physical, emotional, intellectual, professional, social, and spiritual.

Aging within these dimensions of wellness keeps us involved, alert, and enjoying a productive life."

—International Council on Active Aging

Appendix A: Useful Resources

Chapter One

Census Information on 55-plus
www.census.gov/population/www/socdemo/age/
agebyage.html
(866) 758-1060

General Retirement Information
AARP: multitude of resources for those age 50-plus
www.aarp.com

Longevity Calculators
AARP Vitality Compass: http://longevitycalculator.aarp.org

Dr. Thomas Perls of Harvard Medical School:
www.livingto100.com

Dr. Michael Roizen of the Cleveland Clinic:
www.realage.com

National Council on Aging Resources
www.ncoa.org
(202) 479-1200

Retirement Living Options
Resources for seeking housing options in retirement
communities
www.retirementliving.com
www.erickson.com

Social Security Information

Calculate your benefits and find out general information on retirement and Social Security.

www.ssa.gov/retirement

(800) 772-1213

Tai Chi for Health Purposes

http://nccam.nih.gov/health/taichi

VIVA!

A high-tech assessment program to determine a person's physical, mental, emotional strengths. Offers recommendations for keeping what you have or maximizing strengths and minimizing weaknesses during aging. Available in Chicago at Monarch Landing and in Springfield, Virginia, at Greenspring (both Erickson Communities). Open to the public for those 55-plus.

Chicago

www.ericksoncommunities.com/mln

(877) 380-0722

Springfield, Virginia

www.ericksoncommunities.com/gsv

(800) 788-0811

Volunteerism in National Community Programs

SeniorCorps: Tapping the rich experience, skills, and talents of the fifty-five-plus population into community service programs nationwide.

www.seniorcorps.org/

(202) 606-5000

See also "Employment Services" under Chapter Five for mentoring positions and "Experience Corps" Chapter Three Resources listing.

Yoga
http://yoga.about.com/od/beginningyoga/a/seniors.htm

Chapter Two

Advance Directives
The American Bar Association site helps you understand what you need to do to create your advance directive individualized for your needs.
www.abanet.org/aging/toolkit/home.html

Caring Connections allows you to print (state by state) your own advance directives, free at www.caringinfo.org/stateaddownload. Or call (800) 658-8898.

Animation of the Effects of Aging on the Body
This site allows you to click on a part of the body, and it will tell you the effects of aging on that part. Always check with your own physician if you have questions.
www.mydr.com.au/default.asp?article=4157

Assistive and Adaptive Technology
Help children and adults with disabilities enhance their lives, increase their independence and productivity, and gain greater social inclusion through the use of leading-edge assistive technology.
www.rehabtool.com/

Ballroom Dancing
www.fredastaire.com for local dance class listings

Check with local senior centers or community associations for dance classes in your area.

To find a complete listing of local senior centers, go to www
.ncoa.org/content.cfm?sectionID=369&detail=2344.

Diabetes Association
Resources, information, diet, and nutrition
www.diabetes.org

Social networking and online resource for people with
diabetes
www.diabeticconnect.com

Disaboom
Social networking and online resources for persons with
disabilities
www.disaboom.com/Marketplace

Fitness Centers
SilverSneakers program can assist in finding fitness centers
geared for fifty-five-plus. www.silversneakers.com

Jokesercise: An attempt to make fitness accessible to everyone and incorporate laughter
http://jokesercise.com

Heart Disease Information and Resources
American Heart Association
www.americanheart.org

Lifestyle: Technology and Self-learning Assistance
SeniorNet provides adults fifty-five and older with information and instruction about computer technologies. Senior-
Net was incorporated in 1990 as an independent nonprofit
organization.
www.seniornet.org

Mall Walking

If you don't live in a community with climate-controlled walkways, you can go to a mall and join a mall walking program, which enhances fitness and provides socialization. For tips on mall walking, check out www.grandtimes.com/Tips_For_Mall.html.

To find a mall in your area with a mall walking program, check with your senior center or the list of malls nationwide at WalkSport, a program that sponsors mall walking in thirty-eight states: www.walksport.com/sites.htm.

Medical Home Care Model

Erickson Health Medical Centers practice this health model.
www.ericksonhealth.com

Erickson Health Medical Center at Howard County Health Park (not part of retirement community, open to 65-plus, accepts Medicare)
Columbia, MD, (410) 910-6810;
http://ericksonhealthmedcenter.com/locationDirections.html

American Academy of Family Physicians
Information and resources
www.aafp.org

Nutrition

Tips on Healthy Eating and Growing Older
www.fda.gov/cdrh/maturityhealthmatters/issue3.html#3

Nutrition and health after fifty; one size does not fit all. A food pyramid that fits your needs can be found at www.mypyramid.gov.

Osteoporosis: Bone Health, Fall Prevention

Information and resources from the National Osteoporosis
Foundation
www.nof.org/

Smoking Cessation Resources

American Heart Association
www.americanheart.org

American Lung Association
www.lungusa.org
(800) LUNGUSA

CDC smoking cessation materials
www.cdc.gov/tobacco/quit_smoking
/cessation/index.htm

Social Capital Groups

A handbook on how to build a social capital group is available at http://concord.sppsr.ucla.edu/concord.pdf.

Social Networking: Finding or Building a Social Network.

Community centers, volunteer groups, and charitable
organizations are all sources of meeting new people (see
resources under those listings). Online resources include
MySpace.com, which now reports that about 40 percent of
its users are in the thirty-five to fifty-four age group; eons.
com promotes networking for fifty-five-plus.

Blogs: boomers, elders and more. Some of the most popular
blogs that allow for discussion, self-help and meeting others
online are:
Time Goes By (fifty-five and older but mostly sixty-five
plus): TimeGoesBy.net

Kay's Thinking Cap (boomers and above):
http://kaysthinkingcap.blogspot.com
Gen(eration) Between (boomers and above): www.gen
between.com/

Stroke Prevention
www.cdc.gov/stroke/prevention.htm

Vitamins and More
The National Institutes of Health's Medline is a great source
of information on vitamins and more.
www.nlm.nih.gov/medlineplus/vitamins.html

Wii Fit Nintendo Game
With the Wii Balance Board, Wii Fit is a fun, easy way to
work up a sweat. Wii Fit games are divided into four categories: balance games, strength training, yoga, and aerobics.
Choose the difficulty and compete with yourself or with others for the best score. The included Wii Balance Board can be
used in other games, and the in-game personal trainer can
set you up with a daily routine. Available wherever video
games are sold.
www.nintendo.com/wiifit

Chapters Three and Four

Alzheimer's Association
www.alz.org/index.asp

Brain Games
Designed to challenge brain function for all ages.
Big Brain Academy and Brain Challenge DS
www.nintendo.com/games

CogniFit
A series of brain games available for Windows-based computers.
www.cognifit.com

PositScience
The PC-based Brain Fitness Program improves the quality and quantity of the information your brain absorbs from your ears.
www.positscience.com/products/brain_fitness_program

Community Services
Resources for several different types of community services for seniors include:
www.seniorcommunity.org
www.where-to-turn.org

Encore and the Purpose Prize
"Encore careers combine personal fulfillment, social impact and continued income, enabling people to put their passion to work for the greater good. Encore aims to engage millions of boomers in encore careers, providing personal fulfillment doing paid work and producing a windfall of human talent to solve society's greatest problems."
http://encore.org; www.purposeprize.org

Experience Corps
Experience Corps, an award-winning national program, engages people over fifty-five in meeting their communities' greatest challenges. Two thousand Experience Corps members tutor and mentor in twenty-three cities across the country, providing literacy coaching, homework help, consistent role models, and committed, caring attention.
www.experiencecorps.org/index.cfm
(202) 478-6190

Foreign Language Instruction: National Sources
Berlitz School
www.berlitz.com

Foreign language courses online
http://education-portal.com/articles/Free_Foreign
_Language_Courses_Online.html

Pets as Companions
Rescue sites and humane shelters; can be searched via
Google.com for local sites. Some sites of interest:
Rescue Senior Dogs: www.arescuemom.org
PetFinder.com: rescue centers by animal type and localities

Square Dancing
There is a national square dancing association to help you
find a local chapter and get started with this fun exercise.
www.nsdcnec.com

Transportation Services for Seniors
www.seniortransportation.net or seniorservices.org

Travel
Elderhostel
Adventures in lifelong learning and traveling for older
adults; nonprofit organization
www.elderhostel.org
(800) 454-5768

Grand Circle Travel
World leader in international travel, adventure, and discovery for American Travelers over fifty—providing impactful
and intercultural experiences that significantly improve the
quality of their lives

www.gct.com/gcc/general/default.aspx?oid=8530
(800) 959-0405

Widows/Widowers

Grief counseling; widow/spouse support

WidowNet.org
Support group for widows/widowers. Established in 1995, it is the first online information and self-help resource for, and by, widows and widowers. Topics covered include grief, bereavement, recovery, and other information helpful to people of all ages, religious backgrounds, and sexual orientations who have suffered the death of a spouse or life partner.

National Institutes of Health—"Mourning the Death of a Spouse"
www.nia.nih.gov/HealthInformation/Publications/spouse.htm

Comprehensive guide for how to organize your finances after the death of a spouse:
www.gofso.com/Premium/LE/19_le_lo/fg/fg-Death_Spouse.html

Chapter Five

Employment Services

AARP offers both a job search engine (http://jobs.aarp.org) and a National Employer Team (www.aarp.org/employer team), which lists employers that are actively recruiting mature workers nationwide.

RetirementJobs.com (www.retirementjobs.com) has more than thirty thousand listings nationwide from companies specifically seeking candidates older than fifty. A combination job board, adviser, and coach for boomers and seniors looking for work.

RetireeWorkforce.com (www.retireeworkforce.com) focuses on the fifty-plus job candidate.

RetiredBrains.com (www.retiredbrains.com) is a resource for older boomers, seniors, retirees, and those about to retire who are looking to find jobs, volunteer opportunities, educational resources and retirement information.

Retirement Jobs Online (www.retirement-jobs-online.com) offers advice about online retirement jobs, helping retirees evaluate the various ways to use the Internet to find work.

Other sites for seniors seeking full- and part-time employment include:
www.seniorjobbank.org
www.workforce50.com
www.seniors4hire.org
www.seniorjobresource.com

YourEncore (www.yourencore.com) seeks to match retired engineers and scientists with companies that need to meet a capacity surge or fill a short-term need. Clients include Fortune 500 firms such as Boeing, Eli Lilly, and Procter & Gamble. Retirees sometimes are brought in as temporary mentors for new hires.

Financial Resources
The Social Security Administration

www.ssa.gov
(800) 772-1213

Cooperative Extension System
Online learning tools and information about personal finance.
www.mymoney.gov
www.extension.org

National Association of Personal Financial Advisors
For help finding a financial advisor—all charge fees.
www.napfa.org
(800) FEE-ONLY

AARP Personal Finances and Planning
www.aarp.org/money

Mutual fund performance
www.morningstar.com
Also available in the reference section of your local library.

Free or Inexpensive Help for Basic Needs
Meals on Wheels
Provides home-delivered meals to those in need.
(703) 548-5558
www.mowaa.org

The Partnership for Prescription Assistance
The Partnership for Prescription Assistance brings together America's pharmaceutical companies, doctors, other health care providers, patient advocacy organizations, and community groups to help qualifying patients who lack prescription coverage get the medicines they need through the public or private program that's right for them.

www.pparx.org
(888) 4PPA-NOW (477-2669)

Benefits CheckUp
Developed and maintained by The National Council on
Aging (NCOA), BenefitsCheckUp is a comprehensive Web-
based service to screen for benefits programs for seniors
with limited income and resources. BenefitsCheckUp finds
federal, state and private benefit programs available to help
you save money on prescription drugs, health care, utilities,
taxes, and more.
www.benefitscheckup.org/before_you_start.cfm?screen
=BenefitsCheckUpRx
www.BenefitsCheckUp.org

Health Insurance Coverage for Seniors
CMS: Centers for Medicare and Medicaid contains information on all aspects of Medicare and Medicaid.
www.cms.hhs.gov/home/medicare.asp

Medicare, Medicare supplemental policies, Medicare savings accounts, and Medicare advantage plans; go to www
.cms.hhs.gov/center/People.asp.

Those looking for information about Medicare health coverage, Medicare Part D (prescription coverage), should
visit http://medicare.gov or call (800) 633-4227, twenty-
four hours a day, seven days a week for assistance. English-
and Spanish-speaking customer service representatives are
available.

PACE: Program for All-Inclusive Care for the Elderly
www.cms.hhs.gov/pace

Veterans Administration health benefits
(877) 222-8387
www1.va.gov/health/index.asp

Life Insurance

To find an insurer in your state:
The Insurance Information Institute
(212) 346-5500
www.iii.org

To check out an insurance company's performance:
Standard & Poor's Insurance Ratings Service
(212) 438-2000
www.standardandpoor.com

To read or order the Federal Citizen Information Center guide to buying life insurance, "What You Should Know about Buying Life Insurance":
(888) 8-PUEBLO
www.pueblo.gsa.gov

Chapter Six

Caregiver Resources

For those needing help for elderly or disabled parents, spouses, or children.

Adult day care
www.eldercare.gov/eldercare/Public/resources/fact_sheets/adult_day.asp
Explanation and locator of adult day care services
(800) 677-1116. Monday through Friday 9:00 a.m. to 8:00 p.m. (ET)

Assisted living

Assisted living is for adults who need help with everyday tasks such as dressing, bathing, eating, or using the bathroom, but don't need full-time nursing care. Some assisted-living facilities are part of retirement communities. Others are near nursing homes, so a person can move easily if needs change. For more information, go to www.nlm.nih.gov/medlineplus/assistedliving.html

The National Center for Assisted Living's Consumer Guide to Assisted Living and Residential Care Facilities
(202) 842-4444 or www.ncal.org/consumer/thinking.htm

The Assisted Living Federation of America's Consumer Checklist
(703) 691-8100
www.alfa.org/public/articles/details.cfm?id=75

The Consumer Consortium on Assisted Living's Checklist of Questions to Ask When Choosing an Assisted Living Facility
(703) 533-8121
www.ccal.org/checklist.html

Children of Aging Parents (CAPS)

Assists caregivers of the elderly with information and referrals, a network of support groups, and publications and programs that promote public awareness of the value and the needs of family caregivers.
(800) 227-7294
www.caps4caregivers.org

Appendix B: Erickson Resources

Erickson Retirement Communities

Erickson Retirement Communities allow you to pursue your passions. You are rich with experience. You are striving to be even better, and you've earned the right to pursue what brings you pleasure rather than just plain earning. Erickson brings these opportunities to your doorstep in one of our many communities. Reconnect in a dynamic social environment that gives you unlimited opportunities to stay actively involved, yet respects and protects your right to quietly enjoy your privacy. Reawaken the sense of community so often lost in the isolation of today's sprawling cities and suburbs. To understand why Erickson full-service communities are an excellent lifestyle choice a smart financial decision, and to find a community near you, visit us online at www.EricksonCommunities.com or call us at 1-800-380-6211.

John and Nancy Erickson founded The Erickson Foundation in 1998 as a private operating foundation that engages in research as well as philanthropy.

The Foundation's research and development program seeks to advance current best practices in positive aging, including active aging and aging in community with choices.

Through partnerships with university-, government-, and business-based experts, the Foundation's intramural investigators strive to accelerate the completion of translational research that yields real-world applications found to be acceptable, effective, feasible, replicable, affordable, and sustainable.

Previously completed foundation investments in the realm of health and wellness on behalf of older persons include programmatic lines of inquiry pertaining to:

- Descriptive characteristics of persons moving into continuing care retirement communities;

- Clinical epidemiology in older-old and oldest-old adults who reside in senior living communities;

- Comparisons of persons who choose to live in senior living communities versus those who do not;

- Effects of physical activity on cognition and mood;

- Sensory aspects of balance control;

- Health and social changes in late life;

- Health services utilization in late life;

- Changes in choice-making re: amenities and services in late life;

- Experimental shingles vaccine trial;

- Technology-aided comprehensive "whole-person" wellness screenings;

- Changes in strengths and assets related to the physical, psychological, and social aspects of "successful" aging;

- Behavioral, social and psychological consequences of falls;

- Falls and fractures risk reduction;

- Bone health screening, education and referral services;

- Effects of diet and nutrition on cardiovascular health in older adults;

- Benefits of restorative care nursing;

- Non-pharmacological approaches to management of mild hypertension;

- Effects of Tai Chi Chuan on balance, lower extremity strength, and fear of falling;

- Cognitive and physical aspects of memory enhancement;

- Wireless prompting of resident re-positioning to prevent skin lesions;

- Benefits of usage of e-mail and Internet on social relationships;

- Effects of kin relations on the psychological well-being of older adults;

- Experimental avian flu vaccine trial;

- Benefits of late-life learning through active discussion;

- Wireless detection of multi-voiding incidents;

- Validation of performance-based screening tools for older drivers;

- Development and pilot-testing of online end-of-life curriculum for licensed nursing personnel at work in long-term care settings;

- Benefits of group exercise by individuals residing in assisted living facilities;

- Experimental cell-based flu vaccine trial;

- Incidence and correlates of chronic back and/or leg pain in older adults;

- Emergence of patterns of group activity participation in adults residing in continuing care retirement communities;

- Acceptability and effects of wellness education focusing on diet and nutrition, physical activity, stress management and memory enhancement;

- Detection of subtle cognitive decline in the home setting;

Ongoing studies include, but are not limited to:

- Validation of survey tool gauging older men's understanding of bone health and disease;

- Effects of classroom-based education for older drivers on their on-the-road performance;

- Evaluation of behavior change as a result of curbside screenings of the "fit" between older driver and vehicle;

- Effects of computer-based training on modules designed to enhance centralized auditory and visual processing;

- Ability to detect cognitive changes through observation of PC keyboard usage;

- Benefits of treadmill and low-intensity exercises among stroke survivors;

- Alternative approaches to cognitive health and wellness;

- Psychological fitness in late life: Living resiliently with happiness, optimism, and gratitude.

The foundation's research and development team is open to new proposals from diverse prospective partners.

Viva! An Erickson Foundation Initiative

Viva! is a long-term comprehensive assessment and research study that offers participants the chance to take part in health and wellness screenings of:

- bone strength
- balance
- leg strength
- physical activity
- blood pressure
- body composition
- mental health
- life satisfaction
- spirituality
- social support
- community use
- caregiver status

Viva! uses a combination of systematic direct observations, structured quantifiable interviews, and safe, low-burden technologies to assess and monitor participants. The results pinpoint addressable risk factors and participants receive recommendations for improvements in identified areas. Viva! is a long-term program, and participants return for follow-up screenings to compare previous results.

The Erickson School of Aging Studies
(http://erickson.umbc.edu)

John Erickson, founder and chairman of Erickson, and Freeman Hrabowski III, president of University of Maryland, Baltimore County, recognized a significant societal shift and answered it with an interdisciplinary education intended to address every phase of aging in America. The Erickson School offers a bachelor of arts in aging services, a master of arts in the management of aging services, and a variety of executive education courses taught by nationally recognized leaders working in the senior housing and care field, the federal government, academia, and other relevant arenas.

To learn more about the educational programs available to undergraduates, graduates, and executives, go to http://erickson.umbc.org. For more about the Center for Aging Studies' recent research and reports, go to http://erickson.umbc.edu/research/center_aging_studies__elderly_care_services_caring.aspx.

Erickson Health

Erickson Health's goal is to provide tools and services designed to maximize older adults' health. Along with on-campus medical centers and specialty medical care, Erickson Health offers the following services:

- To fight fractures and keep older adults fit, Erickson Health focuses on preventive care strategies such as bone density tests, balance and strength training programs, and consumer education.

- For Erickson residents, Erickson Health provides home care and support services, including comprehensive medication management, short-term extended rehabilitation care with Erickson Health's specially trained physical, speech, and occupational therapists, companions/homemakers, personal care assistance, and nursing care management.

- Renaissance Gardens is the state-of-the-art extended care neighborhood staffed by Erickson Health professionals that offers assisted living, short-term rehabilitation, and long-term nursing care. Details about Renaissance Gardens can be found at www.thecareexperts.com.

- Erickson Health offers Erickson Advantage exclusively to Erickson residents. Erickson Advantage is a Medicare Advantage demonstration project administered by Evercare, offered by United HealthCare Insurance Company, a Medicare Advantage organization with a Medicare contract. For more information about Erickson Advantage, visit www.EricksonAdvantage.com.

- To maximize care accuracy, speed, and coordination, Erickson Health staff use an electronic medical records system that is 100 percent implemented throughout all Erickson communities, including the on-campus medical centers, rehabilitation services, assisted living facilities, long-term care venues, home care services, and emergency medical services. Erickson Health also has electronic Health Information Exchanges in place with local hospitals and specialty practices.

Retirement Living TV

Retirement Living TV's (RLTV) mission is to inform, involve, and inspire viewers and change the world's attitudes, images, and perceptions about aging. RLTV believes television is a promising source for generating positive images of older individuals. Programming provides positive models for older viewers enhancing individuals' sense of control over their lives and their ability to overcome challenges. For more information about program schedules, or to watch clips and participate in interactive forums and games, go to http://rl.tv.

Bibliography

Chapter One

Artificial pacemaker (definition). Online MedicineNet. www. medterms.com/script/main/art.asp?articlekey=7475 (accessed September 27, 2008).

Bard, Terry. Harvard Medical School. Boston, MA. Interview, June 14, 2008.

Bard, Terry. Clinic office. Newton, MA. Interview, July 9, 2008.

DeLong, Thomas. Lecture: "Managing Human Capital." Harvard Business School, Aldrich Hall, September 2005.

Dutko Research Group (sponsored by Erickson government affairs department). "What You Don't Know About Older Americans Can Hurt You" Report. Quantitative survey, administered June 26–July 1, 2006.

Hayflick, Leonard. *How and Why We Age*. New York: Ballantine Books, 1996.

Hillsdon, Melvyn M., Eric J. Brunner, Jack M. Guralnik, and Dr. Michael G. Marmot. "Prospective Study of Physical Activity and Physical Function in Early Old Age." *American Journal of Preventive Medicine*, 28.3 (2005): 245–250.

Idler, Ellen L., and Yael Benyamini. "Self-Rated Health and Mortality: A Review of Twenty-Seven Community Studies." *Journal of Health and Social Behavior*, 38 (1997): 21–37.

Lawrence, Pervin, and John Olive. *Handbook of Personality: Theory and Research, 2nd Edition*. New York: The Guilford Press, 2001.

Machlin, Steven, Joel Cohen, and Karen Beauregard. "Health Care Expenses for Adults with Chronic Conditions, 2005." Medicare Expenditure Panel Survey and Agency for Healthcare Research and Quality Report, May 2008. www.meps.ahrq.gov/mepsweb/data_files/publications/st203/stat203.pdf (accessed October 2, 2008).

Partnership for Solutions. *Chronic Conditions: Making the Case for Ongoing Care*. Baltimore: Johns Hopkins University Press, 2002.

Peterson, Christopher, Steven Maier, and Martin Seligman. *Learned Helplessness: A Theory for the Age of Personal Control*. New York: Oxford University Press, 1995.

Reeves, Matthew. "Healthy Lifestyle Characteristics Among Adults in the United States, 2000." *Archives of Internal Medicine* (April 25, 2005): 165, 854–857.

Seligman, Martin. *Learned Optimism: How to Change Your Mind and Your Life.* New York: Free Press/Simon and Schuster, March 1998.

Social Security and Medicare Boards of Trustees. Trustee Report Summary: A Summary of the 2008 Annual Reports, April 2008. www .ssa.gov/OACT/TRSUM/index.html (accessed October 6, 2008).

Sorkin, John. Lecture: "Biology of Aging." Baltimore: Johns Hopkins University, Wolff Building, November 2006.

U.S. Census Bureau. National Vital Statistics Report: Deaths, Preliminary Data for 2000. 49.12: 23–190.

U.S. Census Bureau. National Vital Statistics Report: Life Expectancy at Birth, by Race and Sex, Selected Years 1929–98.

U.S. Census Bureau. Press Release. April 19, 2002. www.census .gov/Press-Release/www/releases/archives/facts_for_features_ special_editions/000807.html (accessed September 27, 2008).

U.S. Census Bureau. Press Release. May 1, 2008. www.census .gov/Press-Release/www/releases/archives/population/011910. html (accessed September 27, 2008).

Ward, Elizabeth. "Lifestyle, Not Genes, Offers Best Hope of Living Healthier, Longer." *Environmental Nutrition,* April, 2002. http://findarticles.com/p/articles/mi_m0854/is_/ai_n18614124 (accessed September 26, 2008).

Yang, Yang. "Social Inequalities in Happiness in the United States, 1972–2004: An Age-Period-Cohort Analysis." *American Sociological Review,* 73.2 (2008): 4–226.

Chapter Two

Administration on Aging. U.S. Department of Health and Human Services. *A Profile of Older Americans,* 2006.

Arking, Robert. *Biology of Aging: Observations and Principles, 3rd Edition.* New York: Oxford University Press, 2006.

Asimov, Isaac. *The Human Body, and the Human Brain.* New York: Random House, 1985.

Blendon, Robert J., Cathy Schoen, Catherine DesRoches, Robin Osborn, and Kinga Zapert. "Common Concerns Amid Diverse Systems: Health Care Experiences in Five Countries." *Health Affairs*, 2.3 (2003): 106–121.

Brody, Jane. "Preserving a Fundamental Sense: Balance." *The New York Times.* www.nytimes.com/2008/01/08/health/08brod.html?_r=1&oref=slogin (accessed September 27, 2008).

Coppin, Antonia K., Luigi Ferrucci, Fulvio Lauretani, Caroline Phillips, Miran Chang, Stefania Bandinelli, and Jack M. Guralnik. "Low Socioeconomic Status and Disability in Old Age: Evidence from the InChianti Study for the Mediating Role of Physiological Impairments." *The Journals of Gerontology Series A: Biological Sciences and Medical Sciences*, 61 (2006): 86–91.

Dorr, D., A. Wilcox, C. Brunker, R. Burdon, and S. Donnelly. "The Effect of Technology-supported, Multidisease Care Management on the Mortality and Hospitalization of Seniors." *Journal of the American Geriatric Society*, 56 (2008): 2195–2202.

Fischer, W., A. Sirevaag, S. J. Wiegand, R. M. Lindsay, and A. Björklund. "Reversal of Spatial Memory Impairments in Aged Rats by Nerve Growth Factor and Neurotrophins 3 and 4/5 but Not by Brain-derived Neurotrophic Factor." *Proceedings of the National Academy of Sciences.* 91.18 (1994): 8607–8611.

Gustavsson P., L. Alfredsson, H. Brunnberg, N. Hammar, R. Jakobsson, C. Reuterwall, and P. Ostlin. "Myocardial Infarction Among Male Bus, Taxi, and Lorry Drivers in Middle Sweden." *Journal of Occupational and Environmental Medicine.*, 53 (1996): 235–240.

Haffner, Steven M., Seppo Lehto, Tapani Rönnemaa, Kalevi Pyörälä, and Markku Laakso. "Mortality from Coronary Heart Disease in Subjects with Type 2 Diabetes and in Nondiabetic Subjects with and without Prior Myocardial Infarction." *New England Journal of Medicine*, 339.4 (1998): 229–234.

Hayflick, Leonard. *How and Why We Age.* New York: Ballantine Books, 1996.

Hewitt Associates. "Medicare's New Tack Is to Push Prevention." www.hewittassociates.com/Intl/NA/en-US/KnowledgeCenter/HRNews/NewsDetail.aspx?cid=83742164 (accessed September 27, 2008).

Horsley, Shelton J. "On the Use of Olive Oil in Blood-Vessel Suturing."*Annals of Surgery,* 67 (1918): 468–470.

Janssen, Wim G. M., Hans B. J. Bussmann, and Henk J. Stam. "Determinants of the Sit-to-Stand Movement: A Review." *Physical Therapy,* 82 (2002): 866–879.

Koster, Annemarie, Michael F. Leitzmann, Arthur Schatzkin, Traci Mouw, Kenneth F. Adams, Jacques Th. M. van Eijk, Albert R. Hollenbeck, and Tamara B. Harris. "Waist Circumference and Mortality." *American Journal of Epidemiology,* 167.12 (2008): 1465–1475.

Lieberman, Shari. *The Real Vitamin and Mineral Book: Using Supplements for Optimum Health.* New York: Avery Press, 1990.

Martínez-González, Miguel Ángel, C. de la Fuente-Arrillaga, J. M. Nunez-Cordoba, F. J. Basterra-Gortari, J. J. Beunza, Z. Vazquez, S. Benito, A. Tortosa, M. Bes-Rastrollo. "Adherence to Mediterranean Diet and Risk of Developing Diabetes: Prospective Cohort Study." *British Medical Journal,* 336 (2008): 1348–1351.

Moffat, Marilyn and Carole B. Lewis. *Age-Defying Fitness: Making the Most of Your Body for the Rest of Your Life.* Atlanta: Peachtree Publishers, 2006.

National Center for Injury Prevention and Control, Division of Unintentional Injury Prevention, Centers for Disease Control and Prevention. "Preventing Falls Among Older Adults." www.cdc.gov/ncipc/duip/preventadultfalls.htm (accessed September 28, 2008).

Parker-Pope, Tara. "How Does Your Waist Measure Up?" *New York Times,* http://well.blogs.nytimes.com/2008/06/13/how-does-your-waist-measure-up/ (accessed September 28, 2008).

Reinberg, Steven. "Most Older Americans Living Longer and Better." *BusinessWeek,* www.businessweek.com/lifestyle/content/healthday/613967.html?chan=search (accessed September 17, 2008).

Reinboth, Michael and Joan Duda. "Perceived Motivational Climate, Need Satisfaction and Indices of Well-being in Team Sports: A Longitudinal Perspective." *Psychology of Sport and Exercise,* 7.3 (2003): 269–286.

Rosengre, Annika, Karen Anderson, and Lars Wilhelmsen. "Risk of Coronary Heart Disease in Middle-Aged Male Bus and Tram Drivers Compared to Men in Other Occupations: A Prospective Study." *International Journal of Epidemiology,* 20.1: 82–87.

Ruano, J., J. Lopez-Miranda, F. Fuentes, J. Moreno, C. Bellido, P. Perez-Martinez, A. Lozano, P. Gómez, Y. Jiménez, and F. Pérez Jiménez. "Phenolic Content of Virgin Olive Oil Improves Ischemic Reactive Hyperemia in Hypercholesterolemic Patients." *Journal of the American College of Cardiology*, 46.10 (2005): 1864–1868.

Trecroci, Daniel. "Why People Quit Exercising." *Diabetes Health*, published 2001. www.diabeteshealth.com/read/2006/11/01/2150. html (accessed September 28, 2008).

Wischnowsky, Dave. "Wii Bowling Knocks over Retirement Home." *Chicago Tribune*, www.chicagotribune.com/news/local/chi-070216nintendo,0,2755896.story (accessed September 27, 2008).

Wurman, Richard. *Understanding Healthcare*. Newport, Rhode Island: TOP, 2004.

Chapter Three

Abbott, Robert D., Lon R. White, G. Webster Ross, Kamal H. Masaki, J. David Curb, and Helen Petrovitch. "Walking and Dementia in Physically Capable Elderly Men." *Journal of the American Medical Association*, 292 (2004): 1447–1453.

Basak, C., W. Boot, M. Voss, and A. Kramer. "Can Training in a Real-time Strategy Video Game Attenuate Cognitive Decline in Older Adults?" *Psychology and Aging*, 23 (2008): 765–777.

Benedict, Ralph H. B., David Schretlen, Lowell Groninger, and Jason Brandt. "Hopkins Verbal Learning Test—Revised: Normative Data and Analysis of Inter-Form and Test-Retest Reliability." *The Clinical Neuropsychologist*, 12.1 (February 1998): 43–55.

Brandt, Jason. "The Hopkins Verbal Learning Test: Development of a New Memory Test with Six Equivalent Forms." *The Clinical Neuropsychologist*, 5.2 (1991): 125–142.

Carlson, Michelle. Lecture: Experience Corps and Brain Scans of Participants. Mental Health in Later Life. Johns Hopkins University, April 2007.

Carmichael, Mary. "Stronger, Faster, Smarter." *Newsweek*, March 26, 2007. www.newsweek.com/id/36056 (accessed September 28, 2008).

Costacou, T., C. Bamia, P. Ferrari, E. Riboli, D. Trichopoulos, and A. Trichopoulou. "Tracing the Mediterranean Diet through Principal Components and Cluster Analyses in the Greek Population." *European Journal of Clinical Nutrition*, 57 (2003): 1378–1385.

Greene, Kelly. "Putting Brain Exercises to the Test." *Wall Street Journal*, February 3, 2007.

Jorm, Anthony F. "History of Depression as a Risk Factor for Dementia: An Updated Review." *Journal of Psychiatry*, 35.6: 776–781.

Kessing, L. V., and P. K. Andersen. "Does the Risk of Developing Dementia Increase with the Number of Episodes in Patients with Depressive Disorder and in Patients with Bipolar Disorder?" *Journal of Neurology, Neurosurgery and Psychiatry*, 75 (2004): 1662–1666.

Lautenschlager, Nicola T., Kay L. Cox, Leon Flicker, M.B.B.S, Jonathan K. Foster, D. Phil, Frank M. van Bockxmeer, Jianguo Xiao, Kathryn R. Greenop, and Osvaldo P. Almeida. "Effect of Physical Activity on Cognitive Function in Older Adults at Risk for Alzheimer Disease: A Randomized Trial." *Journal of the American Medical Association*, 300.9 (2008): 1027–1037.

Luchsinger, Jose A., Ming-Xin Tang, Yaakov Stern, Steven Shea, and Richard Mayeux. "Diabetes Mellitus and Risk of Alzheimer's Disease and Dementia with Stroke in a Multiethnic Cohort." *American Journal of Epidemiology*, 154.7: 635–641.

Mahncke, H.W., A. Bronstone, and M. M. Merzenich. "Brain Plasticity and Functional Losses in the Aged: Scientific Bases for a Novel Intervention." *Progressive Brain Research*, 157 (2006): 81–109.

Marottoli, Richard A., Heather Allore, Katy L. B. Araujo, Lynne P. Iannone, M.S., Denise Acampora, Margaret Gottschalk, PT, Peter Charpentier, Stanislav Kasl, and Peter Peduzzi. "A Randomized Trial of a Physical Conditioning Program to Enhance the Driving Performance of Older Persons." *Society of General Internal Medicine*, 22 (2007): 590–597.

Moore, B. C., and R.W. Peters. "Pitch Discrimination and Phase Sensitivity in Young and Elderly Subjects and Its Relationship to Frequency Selectivity." *Journal of the Acoustical Society of America.*, 91.5 (May 1992): 2881–2893.

Morrison, J. D., and C. McGrath. "Assessment of the Optical Contributions to the Age-related Deterioration in Vision." *Quarterly Journal of Experimental Physiology*, 70.2 (April 1985): 249–269.

Olincy, A., R. G. Ross, D. A. Youngd, R. Freedman. "Age Diminishes Performance on an Antisaccade Eye Movement Task." *Neurobiology of Aging*, 18.5 (Sep-Oct 1997): 483–489.

Schneider, B. A., and M. K. Pichora-Fuller. "Implications of Perceptual Deterioration for Cognitive Aging Research." In: Craik F. I. M. and T. A. Salthouse, eds. *The Handbook of Aging and Cognition.* Mahwah, NJ: Lawrence Erlbaum Associates, 2000: 155–219.

Sofi, Francesco, Francesca Cesari, Rosanna Abbate, Gian Franco Gensini, and Alessandro Casini. "Adherence to Mediterranean Diet and Health Status: Meta-analysis." *British Medical Journal*, 337 (2008): 1344.

Sorkin, John (University of Maryland). Lecture: "Biology of Aging." Baltimore, Johns Hopkins University, Wolff Building, November 2006.

Tan, Erwin, Qian-Li Xue, Tao Li, Michelle Carlson, and Linda Fried. "Volunteering: A Physical Activity Intervention for Older Adults—The Experience Corps Program in Baltimore." *Journal of Urban Health*, 83.5 (Sep. 2006): 954–969.

U.S. Department of Health and Human Services. Physical Activity and Health: A Report of the Surgeon General. Atlanta: Centers for Disease Control and Prevention (CDC), National Center for Chronic Disease Prevention and Health Promotion, 1996. www.cdc.gov/nccdphp/sgr/sgr.htm (accessed September 29, 2008).

Verghese, Joe, Richard B. Lipton, Mindy J. Katz, Charles B. Hall, Carol A. Derby, Gail Kuslansky, Anne F. Ambrose, Martin Sliwinski, and Herman Buschke. "Leisure Activities and the Risk of Dementia in the Elderly." *New England Journal of Medicine*, 348.25 (2003): 2508-2516.

Weuve, Jennifer, Jae Hee Kang, JoAnn E. Manson, Monique M. B. Breteler, James H. Ware, and Francine Grodstein . "Physical Activity, Including Walking, and Cognitive Function in Older Women." *Journal of the American Medical Association*, 292 (2004): 1454–1461.

Willis, Sherry L., Sharon L. Tennstedt, Michael Marsiske, Karlene Ball, Jeffrey Elias, Kathy Mann Koepke, John N. Morris, George W. Rebok, Frederick W. Unverzagt, Anne M. Stoddard, and Elizabeth Wright. "Long-term Effects of Cognitive Training on Everyday Functional Outcomes in Older Adults." *Journal of the American Medical Association*, 296.23 (December 20, 2006).

Woodruff-Pak, D. S. "Neural Plasticity as a Substrate for Cognitive Adaptation in Adulthood and Aging." In: Cerella J., J. Rybash, W. Hover, and M. L. Commons, eds. *Adult Information Processing: Limits on Loss.* San Diego: Academic Press, 1993.

Chapter Four

Abtouche, Susan L. "Civic Engagement: Principles and Issues in a Retirement Community." Chestnut Hill College GAHS 599—Special Project, Dr. Green, December 6, 2007.

"Challenging Long-Held Assumptions About Workplace Friendships" (book review). WP Carey Knowledge, http://knowledge. wpcarey.asu.edu/article.cfm?articleid=1616 (accessed November 1, 2008).

Christakis, Nicholas A., and Paul D. Allison. "Mortality after the Hospitalization of a Spouse." *New England Journal of Medicine,* 354.7 (February 16, 2006): 719–730.

Damasio, Antonio R., Thomas J. Grabowski, Antoine Bechara, Hanna Damasio, Laura L. B. Ponto, Josef Parvizi, and Richard D. Hichwa. "Subcortical and Cortical Brain Activity During the Feeling of Self-generated Emotions." *Nature Neuroscience,* 3 (2000): 1049– 1056.

Duke University. Press Release. "Activation of Brain Region Predicts Altruism." Duke Medicine News and Communications, www .dukehealth.org/HealthLibrary/News/9998 (accessed November 1, 2008).

Encore nonprofit Web site. www.encore.org/news/encore_ campaign (accessed November 4, 2008).

Estruch, Ramón, M.A. Martínez-González, D. Corella, J. Salas-Salvadó, V. Ruiz-Gutiérrez, M. I. Covas, M. Fiol, E. Gómez-Gracia, M. C. López-Sabater, E. Vinyoles, F. Arós, M. Conde, C. Lahoz, J. Lapetra, G. Sáez, and E. Ros. "Effects of a Mediterranean-style Diet on Cardiovascular Risk Factors: A Randomized Trial." *Annals of Internal Medicine,* 4.145 (2006): 1–11.

Kouvonen, Anne, Tuula Oksanen, Jussi Vahtera, Mai Stafford, Richard Wilkinson, Justine Schneider, Ari Väänänen, Marianna Virtanen, Sara J. Cox, Jaana Pentti, Marko Elovainio, and Mika Kivimäki. "Low Workplace Social Capital as a Predictor of Depression." *American Journal of Epidemiology,* 167 (2008): 1143–1151.

Kristof, Nicholas D. "Geezers Doing Good." *The New York Times,* July 20, 2008, Opinions section, online edition. www.nytimes.com/2008/07/20/opinion/20kristof.html?_r=2&oref=slogin&oref=slogin (accessed November 4, 2008).

Luoh, Ming-Ching, and A. Regula Herzog. "Individual Consequences of Volunteer and Paid Work in Old Age: Health and Mortality." *Journal of Health and Social Behavior,* 43.4 (December 2002): 490–509.

Morgan, K., H. M. Dallosso, and S. B. J. Ebrahim. "A Brief Self-report Scale for Assessing Personal Engagement in the Elderly." In Butler, A. ed. *Ageing: Recent Advances and Creative Responses.* London: Croam Helm, 1985.

Older Americans 2008: Key Indicators of Well-Being. Federal Interagency on Aging Related Statistics. Washington, DC: U.S. Government Printing Office, March 2008.

Requena, Felix. "Social Capital, Satisfaction and Quality of Life in the Workplace." *Social Indicators Research,* 61.3 (2003): 331–360.

Todorova, Aleksandra. "Switching Careers at 50, Boomers Look for Fulfillment." *Smart Money,* September 28, 2007, www.smart-money.com/personal-finance/retirement/switching-careers-at-50-boomers-look-for-fulfillment-21896/ (accessed November 10, 2008).

University of California. Press Release. "Brain's Amygdala Region Acts as Danger Detector," University of California newsroom online, June 20, 2001, www.universityofcalifornia.edu/news/article/3364 (accessed October 12, 2008).

University of Pennsylvania Press Release. "Hospitalization or Death of Elderly Spouse Substantially Affects Husband or Wife's Mortality." University of Pennsylvania Office of University Communications, February 15, 2006, www.upenn.edu/pennnews/article.php?id=912 (accessed November 1, 2008).

U.S. Administration on Aging, University of Missouri, and National Science Foundation. "Using Technology to Enhance Aging in Place." Proceedings presented at International Conference on Smart Homes and Health Telematics, 2008.

Wolff, Jennifer L., and Debra L. Roter. "Hidden in Plain Sight: Medical Visit Companions as a Resource for Vulnerable Older Adults." *Archives of Internal Medicine,* 168.13 (2008): 1409–1415.

Yang, Yang. "Social Inequalities in Happiness in the United States, 1972–2004: An Age-Period-Cohort Analysis." *American Sociological Review,* 73.2 (2008): 204–226.

Chapter Five

Barrie, Margie. "The odds are . . . you'll need LTC." *Senior Market Advisor,* September 1, 2007. www.seniormarketadvisor.com/r/smaMag/d/contentFocus/?adcID=1fc0f85733332a7d21d0ff4f4268f06d (accessed November 7, 2008).

Centers for Medicare and Medicaid Services, www.medicare.gov (accessed November 1, 2008).

Cohen, Andrea. Newton, MA. Interview, June 12, 2008.

Matthews, Joseph L., and Dorothy Matthews-Berman. *Social Security, Medicare & Government Pensions: Get the Most Out of Your Retirement & Medical Pensions.* Berkeley, CA: NOLO Publishing, 2008.

Social Security Administration, www.ssa.gov (accessed November 1, 2008).

Tomkiel, Stanley. *The Social Security Benefits Handbook,* 5th Edition. Naperville, IL: Sphinx Publishing, 2008.

Zaleznick, Steve. Interview, Longevity Alliance Office, Washington, DC, May 9, 2008.

Chapter Six

Abtouche, Susan L. "Civic Engagement: Principles and Issues in a Retirement Community." Special project paper for Class GAHS 599, Chestnut Hill College, 2007.

Ameriprise Financial. Press Release. "The New Retirement Mindscape." January 23, 2006. www.ameriprise.com/amp/global/sitelets/dreambook/pr-home.asp (accessed November 1, 2008).

Atchley, R. C., and A. S. Barusch. *Social Forces and Aging: An Introduction to Social Gerontology.* Belmont, MA: Wadsworth Thomson, 2004.

Brown, Kathi W. "Staying Ahead of the Curve 2003: The AARP Working in Retirement Study." AARP.

Butler, Robert N. "Age-ism: Another Form of Bigotry." *The Gerontologist,* 9 (1969): 243–246.

Greene, Kelly. "Report Finds Heavier Cost for Caregivers." *Wall Street Journal*, November 20, 2008, http://online.wsj.com/article/SB122715318473143813.html (accessed December 1, 2008).

He, W., M. Sengupta, V. Velkoff, and K. DeBarros. "65+ in the United States." *U.S. Census Bureau, Current Population Reports (2005)*, www.census.gov/prod/2006pubs/p23-209/ (accessed November 20, 2008).

Kleinspehn-Ammerlahn, A., D. Kotter-Grühn, and J. Smith. "Self-perceptions of Aging: Do Subjective Age and Satisfaction with Aging Change During Old Age?" *Journals of Gerontology*, 63 (2008): P377–85.

Korczyk, Sophie. "Who is Ready for Retirement, How Ready, and How Can We Know?" Research Report, AARP (January 2008), www.aarp.org/research/financial/retirementsaving/inb154_income.html (accessed November 20, 2008).

Levya, Becca R., Martin D. Sladeb, and Stanislav V. Kasla. "Longitudinal Benefit of Positive Self-Perceptions of Aging on Functional Health." *Journals of Gerontology Series B: Psychological Sciences and Social Science*, 57(2002): 409–417.

Reilly, S. L. "Transforming Aging: The Civic Engagement of Adults 55+." *Public Policy & Aging Report*, 16 (2006). www.agingsociety.org/agingsociety/publications/public_policy/PPAR_Fall_2006 (accessed November 20, 2008).

Zelinski, E. J. *How to Retire Happy, Wild, and Free.* Berkeley, CA: Ten Speed Press, 2007.

Acknowledgments

Many people were involved in the creation of this book, from broad-brush visionaries to field-tested experts.

We owe huge debts of gratitude to our editor Lara Asher and agents Steve Harris and Michele Martin, who guided us skillfully from start to finish in the book creation process. Steve, if your verisimilitude is ever bottled and sold, we will be your first customers. Michele, the same goes for your creative ideas. Lara, thank you for being a master at working with several cooks in the kitchen.

In addition, a remarkable organization fueled us in the writing of these words.

If John Erickson had not opened Charlestown community in 1983 with the help of his lovely wife, Nancy, and astute family members such as Michael, we could not have accumulated twenty-five years' worth of stories, wisdom, and research to share. We appreciate the vision and encouragement of John, Nancy, and Michael—and now Craig, Scott, and Andrea—in helping to develop this book.

Since 1983, Erickson has grown into a large family of more than 13,000 employees, 22,000 residents, and countless friends and mentors. We discovered the strength and depth of this greater Erickson family when we were able to call nearly any member of it and receive thoughtful, useful advice.

Specifically, Nancy Belle has exceeded the call of family to help lead us when we were lost in book writing. Carla Ulgen has been a fount of knowledge and savvy in helping to keep us out of trouble. Donna Samulowitz helped us stay one step ahead in our thinking, and Tom Neubauer and Deb Doyle gave us impetus in the early stages.

Ron Colasanti as introduced by Rob Bobbitt provided us with many creative food and dining ideas. Kim Jordan graciously offered her expertise and insights on exercise and physical therapy. Chris Miles and Arline Davis amazed us with how easily they could access stories and anecdotes from memory. Dr. Brandwin, as always, had interesting and funny quips to contribute. Joy Kim and Peggy Chalson were lifesavers for their ability to schedule emergency meetings, not to mention their prowess with Microsoft *Office*.

John Parrish and Jean Gaines of the Erickson Foundation lent us their keen intelligence for guidance, content, and advice. Participants in the Erickson Foundation's Viva! research study graciously shared their successes and lessons.

Horace Deets, formerly head of AARP, tapped into his wealth of experience, both personal and professional, to help guide us. Andrea Cohen, CEO of HouseWorks, gave us insight into intentional communities and social entrepreneurship. Steve Zaleznick, CEO of Longevity Alliance, showed us the ins and outs of products that could provide financial security. Larry Minnix, head of AAHSA, the largest industry group, helped us brainstorm ideas, styles, and formats.

We were also fortunate to have academic practitioners offer their advice and comments, including Dr. Terry Bard of Harvard Medical School with his affable anecdotes, and Dr. George Rebok of Johns Hopkins School of Public Health with his world-renowned work in aging and mental health. Harvard-trained M.D. and Ph.D. neuroscientist Jay Chyung helped explain concepts such as brain plasticity and learning.

Most of all, we were extremely lucky to have the input of our retirement community residents, whose stories, life lessons, and jokes inspired the stories used to bring to life the statistics and studies explored in this book. We are an organization that exists to serve our residents, and we feel honored to have so many people who shared their thoughts, suggestions, and advice freely with us, including the following individuals:

Mrs. Brooks
The Churches
Mrs. Clark
The Coulters
Mrs. Cumbie
Dr. Dake
Dr. Feldstein
Mr. Francisco
The Gralleys
"Miss Irene"
The Jaekles
The Kaminskis
Mrs. Keller
Mr. Margosis
Miss Muldoon
Mr. Norton
The Pledgers
The Reynolds
Mr. Riley
The Sklenars
The Taylors
The Tsos
The Westburgs

Index

About the Authors

Mark R. Erickson

Mark Erickson is the chief operating officer/president of health and operations for Erickson, with responsibilities for operations and development of the core senior housing business. He oversees a billion-dollar business that serves 22,000 seniors and 11,000 employees at more than twenty continuing care retirement communities across the country.

Before rejoining Erickson in 2000, Mark spent five years with American Express Consulting Services based in Europe and Asia. He earned a B.A. in English literature at Vanderbilt University and an M.B.A. from the Wharton School at University of Pennsylvania.

Currently, Mark serves as a board member or trustee for the following organizations—the Institute of Notre Dame, Leadership Baltimore County, the executive committee of the American Senior Housing Association, and Catholic Charities.

Matthew J. Narrett, M.D.

Dr. Matthew Narrett is the executive vice president and chief medical officer for Erickson. He is responsible for directing the provision of medical care and the Erickson Health Strategy at all Erickson communities. The medical centers that Dr. Narrett directs are recognized as America's leading geriatric health care facilities.

Prior to his current position and over the course of his sixteen years at Erickson, Dr. Narrett served as senior vice president and chief medical officer, vice president and regional medical director, and medical director for Charlestown, an Erickson community in Baltimore. Before joining

Erickson, he was in private practice in Derry, New Hampshire, where he also served as director of medical quality assurance at Parkland Medical Center. He has extensive experience in adult medicine, having treated thousands of seniors throughout his over twenty-five-year career.

Dr. Narrett holds a B.S. in molecular biochemistry and biophysics, graduating summa cum laude from Yale University. He received his medical degree from Harvard Medical School, Harvard–M.I.T. Division of Health Sciences and Technology. He completed his internship and residency at Beth Israel Hospital in Boston.

He is board certified in internal medicine and holds a certificate of added qualifications in geriatric medicine.

Dr. Narrett currently serves on the Clinical Practice and Models of Care Committee for the American Geriatric Society and the Advisory Board of the Practice Change Fellows Program supported by the Atlantic Philanthropies and the John A. Hartford Foundation. He is also a member of the American College of Physicians and the American Geriatrics Society.

He has spoken on issues affecting seniors in a number of venues including conferences, media events, health leadership summits, and congressional forums.

Jacquelyn Kung

Jacquelyn is a social entrepreneur in the senior living industry. She was formerly associate executive director of Erickson's Greenspring Village, one of the largest retirement communities in Virginia. In 2004, she published an educational guidebook with McGraw-Hill.

Jacquelyn holds an M.B.A. and a B.A. from Harvard University and received her doctorate with a focus on aging studies from the Johns Hopkins School of Public Health.

Lisa Davila

Lisa is a senior health writer for Erickson. She is responsible for writing and editing health-related materials for all Erickson communities.

Lisa holds a B.S. in nursing and an M.S. in medical and science writing from Towson University. She is a member of the American Medical Writers Association.